DATE DUE

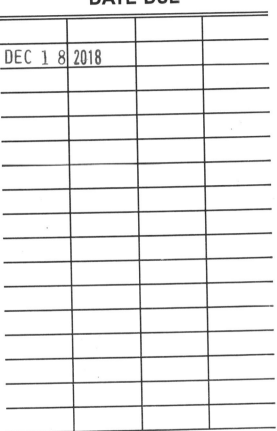

DEC 1 8 2018			

Demco, Inc. 38-293

Asthma Information for Teens

Second Edition

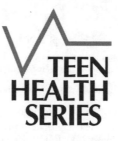

TEEN HEALTH SERIES

Second Edition

Asthma Information for Teens

Health Tips about Managing Asthma and Related Concerns

Including Facts about Asthma Causes, Triggers and Symptoms, Diagnosis, and Treatment

◆

Edited by Kim Wohlenhaus

Omnigraphics

P.O. Box 31-1640, Detroit, MI 48231

Bibliographic Note

Because this page cannot legibly accommodate all the copyright notices, the Bibliographic Note portion of the Preface constitutes an extension of the copyright notice.

Edited by Kim Wohlenhaus

Teen Health Series

Karen Bellenir, *Managing Editor*
David A. Cooke, MD, FACP, *Medical Consultant*
Elizabeth Collins, *Research and Permissions Coordinator*
Cherry Edwards, *Permissions Assistant*
EdIndex, Services for Publishers, *Indexers*

* * *

Omnigraphics, Inc.

Matthew P. Barbour, *Senior Vice President*
Kevin M. Hayes, *Operations Manager*

* * *

Peter E. Ruffner, *Publisher*

Copyright © 2010 Omnigraphics, Inc.

ISBN 978-0-7808-1086-0

Library of Congress Cataloging-in-Publication Data

Asthma information for teens : health tips about managing asthma and related concerns including facts about asthma causes, triggers and symptoms, diagnosis, and treatment / edited by Kim Wohlenhaus. -- 2nd ed.
    p. cm.
  Summary: "Provides basic consumer health information for teens about asthma causes and treatments, controlling triggers, and coping with asthma at home and school. Includes index, resource information and recommendations for further reading"--Provided by publisher.
  Includes bibliographical references and index.
  ISBN 978-0-7808-1086-0 (hardcover : alk. paper) 1. Asthma--Popular works. 2. Teenagers--Diseases--Popular works. I. Wohlenhaus, Kim.

RC591.A818117 2010
616.2'38--dc22

                                                    2009048694

Table of Contents

Part Three: Medications Used To Treat Asthma Symptoms

Part Four: Other Medical Conditions And Asthma

Part Five: Lifestyle Issues In Asthma Management

Part Six: Asthma Research

Part Seven: If You Need Additional Help And Information

Preface

About This Book

According to the Centers for Disease Control and Prevention (CDC), just under seven million U.S. children and adolescents under the age of 18 currently have asthma, and more than four million have had an asthma attack in the past 12 months. Many others have "hidden" or undiagnosed asthma. Although some people may believe that asthma is not serious—that it is just an inconvenience or that the asthma sufferer is simply lazy—this is a misconception. Asthma is a chronic, inflammatory lung disease that cannot be cured or prevented; however, with knowledge and proper medical care, asthma can be successfully managed.

Asthma Information for Teens, Second Edition provides introductory information for teens who have recently received a diagnosis of asthma, and it offers in-depth information for teens who have had experience dealing with asthma since early childhood. It includes information about various forms of asthma, factors that may contribute to the development of asthma, and common asthma triggers, such as pollen, dust mites, mold, tobacco smoke, cockroaches, animal dander, and some chemicals. Commonly used asthma medications and delivery devices are discussed, and lifestyle adjustments used in managing asthma and controlling asthma flares are explained. A section on current asthma-related research is also included, along with a directory of resources and suggestions for teens who would like to read more about asthma.

How To Use This Book

This book is divided into parts and chapters. Parts focus on broad areas of interest; chapters are devoted to single topics within a part.

Part One: Asthma Facts provides an overview of the lungs and respiratory system and explains the various types of asthma, including exercise-induced asthma, nocturnal asthma, and occupational asthma. National and global asthma data are presented, including statistics specifically related to children, young adults, and diverse communities. Risk factors for developing asthma are also discussed.

Part Two: Diagnosing And Managing Asthma explains how doctors diagnose asthma and treat symptoms. Chapters about what a pulmonologist does, when an allergist should be consulted, and what allergy testing entails are included. Methods of monitoring and managing asthma symptoms are covered, including information about how to use a peak flow meter and how to deal with asthma flare-ups.

Part Three: Medications Used To Treat Asthma Symptoms discusses the different types of medicines that are commonly used by asthma sufferers, including anti-IgE treatment, bronchodilators, corticosteroids, cromolyn sodium, montelukast and other leukotriene modifiers, and theophylline. The advantages and side effects of inhaled steroids and dry powder inhalers are discussed, and the use of asthma medication devices is described. The part concludes with information about alternative therapies used for managing asthma.

Part Four: Other Medical Conditions And Asthma provides an overview of medical conditions related to respiratory health and asthma. The connection between allergies and asthma is discussed, and links with such other diseases as chronic obstructive pulmonary disease (COPD), gastroesophageal reflux disease (GERD), coughing, colds and influenza, rhinitis, and sinusitis are explained.

Part Five: Lifestyle Issues In Asthma Management provides information about living with and successfully treating asthma. Partnering with a doctor, developing an asthma action plan, using medicines appropriately, and identifying asthma triggers are all discussed. Chapters in this part also offer tips about good health habits for people with asthma, including exercising, understanding the importance of good nutrition, and avoiding tobacco products. Problems related to treatment plan nonadherence and suggestions for dealing with asthma emergencies are also addressed.

Part Six: Asthma Research includes an overview of the National Asthma Control Program—what is being done to reduce the number of deaths, hospitalizations, emergency department visits, school and work days missed, and limitations on activity due to asthma. It also reports on airborne pollutants, the effects of hormonal fluctuations on asthma control, and newly developed treatments, such as bronchial thermoplasty. Facts about medicines that might aggravate asthma are also presented.

Part Seven: If You Need Additional Help And Information provides a directory of asthma organizations and suggestions for additional reading about asthma and related topics.

Bibliographic Note

This volume contains documents and excerpts from publications issued by the following government agencies: Centers for Disease Control and Prevention; National Cancer Institute; National Digestive Diseases Information Clearinghouse; National Heart, Lung, and Blood Institute; National Institute of Allergy and Infectious Diseases; National Institute of Environmental Health Sciences; U.S. Environmental Protection Agency; and the U.S. Food and Drug Administration.

In addition, this volume contains copyrighted documents and articles produced by the following organizations: A.D.A.M., Inc.; Allergy and Asthma Network Mothers of Asthmatics; American Academy of Allergy, Asthma and Immunology; American Association for Respiratory Care; American College of Allergy, Asthma and Immunology; American College of Chest Physicians; American Lung Association; American Society of Health-System Pharmacists; Asthma and Allergy Foundation of America; Asthma Initiative of Michigan (AIM); Asthma Society of Canada; Canadian Centre for Occupational Health and Safety; Cleveland Clinic Foundation; CMP Medica; Family Allergy and Asthma; Global Initiative for Asthma; HealthCentral Network, Inc.; Morefocus Media, Inc.; Nemours Foundation; New Jersey Department of Health and Senior Services; New York City

Asthma Initiative; Permanente Medical Group, Inc.; ScoutNews, LLC; Texas Medical Center; and the World Health Organization.

The photograph on the front cover is from Creatas Images via Jupiter Images.

Full citation information is provided on the first page of each chapter. Every effort has been made to secure all necessary rights to reprint the copyrighted material. If any omissions have been made, please contact Omnigraphics to make corrections for future editions.

Acknowledgements

In addition to the organizations listed above, special thanks are due to the *Teen Health Series* research and permissions coordinator, Elizabeth Collins, and to its managing editor, Karen Bellenir.

About The *Teen Health Series*

At the request of librarians serving today's young adults, the *Teen Health Series* was developed as a specially focused set of volumes within Omnigraphics' *Health Reference Series*. Each volume deals comprehensively with a topic selected according to the needs and interests of people in middle school and high school.

Teens seeking preventive guidance, information about disease warning signs, medical statistics, and risk factors for health problems will find answers to their questions in the *Teen Health Series*. The *Series*, however, is not intended to serve as a tool for diagnosing illness, in prescribing treatments, or as a substitute for the physician/patient relationship. All people concerned about medical symptoms or the possibility of disease are encouraged to seek professional care from an appropriate health care provider.

If there is a topic you would like to see addressed in a future volume of the *Teen Health Series*, please write to:

Editor
Teen Health Series
Omnigraphics, Inc.
P.O. Box 31-1640
Detroit, MI 48231

A Note About Spelling And Style

Teen Health Series editors use *Stedman's Medical Dictionary* as an authority for questions related to the spelling of medical terms and the *Chicago Manual of Style* for questions related to grammatical structures, punctuation, and other editorial concerns. Consistent adherence is not always possible, however, because the individual volumes within the *Series* include many documents from a wide variety of different producers and copyright holders, and the editor's primary goal is to present material from each source as accurately as is possible following the terms specified by each document's producer. This sometimes means that information in different chapters or sections may follow other guidelines and alternate spelling authorities. For example, occasionally a copyright holder may require that eponymous terms be shown in possessive forms (Crohn's disease *vs.* Crohn disease) or that British spelling norms be retained (leukaemia *vs.* leukemia).

Locating Information Within The *Teen Health Series*

The *Teen Health Series* contains a wealth of information about a wide variety of medical topics. As the *Series* continues to grow in size and scope, locating the precise information needed by a specific student may become more challenging. To address this concern, information about books within the *Teen Health Series* is included in *A Contents Guide to the Health Reference Series*. The *Contents Guide* presents an extensive list of more than 15,000 diseases, treatments, and other topics of general interest compiled from the Tables of Contents and major index headings from the books of the *Teen Health Series* and *Health Reference Series*. To access *A Contents Guide to the Health Reference Series*, visit www.healthreferenceseries.com.

Our Advisory Board

We would like to thank the following advisory board members for providing guidance to the development of this *Series*:

Dr. Lynda Baker, Associate Professor of Library and Information Science, Wayne State University, Detroit, MI

Nancy Bulgarelli, William Beaumont Hospital Library, Royal Oak, MI

Karen Imarisio, Bloomfield Township Public Library, Bloomfield Township, MI

Karen Morgan, Mardigian Library, University of Michigan-Dearborn, Dearborn, MI

Rosemary Orlando, St. Clair Shores Public Library, St. Clair Shores, MI

Medical Consultant

Medical consultation services are provided to the *Teen Health Series* editors by David A. Cooke, MD, FACP. Dr. Cooke is a graduate of Brandeis University, and he received his M.D. degree from the University of Michigan. He completed residency training at the University of Wisconsin Hospital and Clinics. He is board-certified in internal medicine. Dr. Cooke currently works as part of the University of Michigan Health System and practices in Ann Arbor, MI. In his free time, he enjoys writing, science fiction, and spending time with his family.

Part One
Asthma Facts

Chapter 1

The Lungs And Respiratory System

Whether you're wide awake and getting ready for a big date or asleep during your most snooze-worthy afternoon class, you don't have to think about breathing. It's so important to life that it happens automatically. If you didn't breathe, you couldn't live.

What Are The Lungs And Respiratory System And What Do They Do?

Each day we breathe about 20,000 times. All of this breathing couldn't happen without help from the respiratory system, which includes the nose, throat, voice box, windpipe, and lungs. With each breath, you take in air through your nostrils and mouth, and your lungs fill up and empty out. As air is inhaled, the mucous membranes of the nose and mouth warm and humidify the air.

Although we can't see it, the air we breathe is made up of several gases. Oxygen is the most important for keeping us alive because body cells need it for energy and growth. Without oxygen, the body's cells would die.

About This Chapter: Text in this chapter is from "Lungs and Respiratory System," April 2007, reprinted with permission from www.kidshealth.org. Copyright © 2007 The Nemours Foundation. This information was provided by KidsHealth, one of the largest resources online for medically reviewed health information written for parents, kids, and teens. For more articles like this one, visit www.KidsHealth.org, or www.TeensHealth.org.

Carbon dioxide is the waste gas that is produced when carbon is combined with oxygen as part of the body's energy-making processes. The lungs and respiratory system allow oxygen in the air to be taken into the body, while also enabling the body to get rid of carbon dioxide in the air breathed out.

Respiration is the term for the exchange of oxygen from the environment for carbon dioxide from the body's cells. The process of taking air into the lungs is called inhalation or inspiration, and the process of breathing it out is called exhalation or expiration.

Even if the air you breathe is dirty or polluted, your respiratory system filters out foreign matter and organisms that enter through the nose and mouth. Pollutants are breathed or coughed out, destroyed by digestive juices, or eaten by macrophages, a type of blood cell that patrols the body looking for germs to destroy.

> ### ♣ It's A Fact!!
> ### How fast is a sneeze?
>
> If your sneeze were a car, it would get a ticket for speeding. When you sneeze, particles fly out of your nose at 100 miles per hour. A sneeze is the body's way of getting rid of something that's irritating the nose. Your nose feels a tickle and the sneeze center in your brain responds by coordinating muscles in your belly, chest, and diaphragm to sneeze out the irritant.
>
> Source: © 2007 Nemours Foundation.

Tiny hairs called cilia (pronounced: sih-lee-uh) protect the nasal passageways and other parts of the respiratory tract, filtering out dust and other particles that enter the nose with the breathed air. As air is inhaled, the cilia move back and forth, pushing any foreign matter (like dust) either toward the nostrils, where it is blown out, or toward the pharynx, where it travels through the digestive system and out with the rest of the body's waste.

The two openings of the airway (the nasal cavity and the mouth) meet at the pharynx (pronounced: far-inks), or throat, at the back of the nose and mouth. The pharynx is part of the digestive system as well as the respiratory system because it carries both food and air. At the bottom of the pharynx, the pathway for both food and air divides in two. One passageway is for food (the esophagus, pronounced: ih-sah-fuh-gus, which leads to the stomach) and the other for air. The epiglottis (pronounced: eh-pih-glah-tus), a small flap of tissue, covers the air-only passage when we swallow, keeping food and liquid from going into our lungs.

The larynx (pronounced: lar-inks), or voice box, is the uppermost part of the air-only passage. This short tube contains a pair of vocal cords, which vibrate to make sounds. The trachea (pronounced: tray-kee-uh), or windpipe, extends downward from the base of the larynx. It lies partly in the neck and partly in the chest cavity. The walls of the trachea are strengthened by stiff rings of cartilage to keep it open so air can flow through on its way to

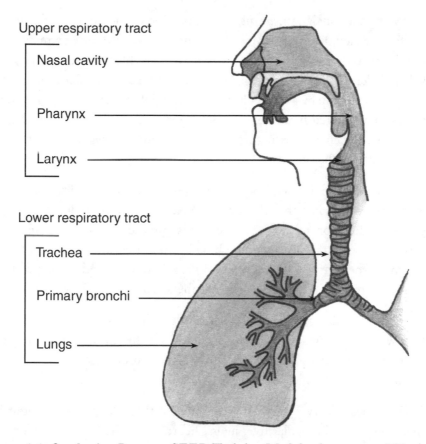

Figure 1.1. Conducting Passages. SEER Training Module, Anatomy and Physiology, National Cancer Institute. Image re-drawn for Omnigraphics by Alison DeKleine.

the lungs. The trachea is also lined with cilia, which sweep fluids and foreign particles out of the airway so that they stay out of the lungs.

At its bottom end, the trachea divides into left and right air tubes called bronchi (pronounced: brahn-ky), which connect to the lungs. Within the lungs, the bronchi branch into smaller bronchi and even smaller tubes called bronchioles (pronounced: brahn-kee-olz). Bronchioles, which are as thin as a strand of hair, end in tiny air sacs called alveoli (pronounced: al-vee-oh-lie). Each of us has hundreds of millions of alveoli in our lungs—enough to cover a tennis court if they were spread out on the ground. The alveoli are where the exchange of oxygen and carbon dioxide takes place.

With each inhalation, air fills a large portion of the millions of alveoli. In a process called diffusion (pronounced: dih-fyoo-zhun), oxygen moves from the alveoli to the blood through the capillaries (tiny blood vessels, pronounced: kah-puh-ler-eez) that line the alveolar walls. Once in the bloodstream, oxygen gets picked up by a molecule called hemoglobin (pronounced: hee-muh-glo-bun) in the red blood cells. This oxygen-rich blood then flows back to the heart, which pumps it through the arteries to oxygen-hungry tissues throughout the body.

In the tiny capillaries of the body tissues, oxygen is freed from the hemoglobin and moves into the cells. Carbon dioxide, which is produced during the process of diffusion, moves out of these cells into the capillaries, where most of it is dissolved in the plasma of the blood. Blood rich in carbon dioxide then returns to the heart via the veins. From the heart, this blood is pumped to the lungs, where carbon dioxide passes into the alveoli to be exhaled.

The lungs also contain elastic tissues that allow them to inflate and deflate without losing shape and are encased by a thin lining called the pleura (pronounced: plur-uh). This network of alveoli, bronchioles, and bronchi is known as the bronchial tree.

The chest cavity, or thorax (pronounced: thor-aks), is the airtight box that houses the bronchial tree, lungs, heart, and other structures. The top and sides of the thorax are formed by the ribs and attached muscles, and the bottom by a large muscle called the diaphragm. The chest walls form a protective cage around the lungs and other contents of the chest cavity.

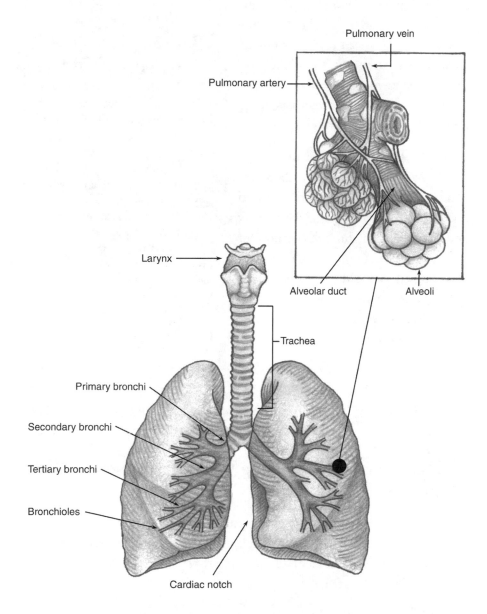

Figure 1.2. *Bronchi, Bronchial Tree, and Lungs. SEER Training Module, Anatomy and Physiology, National Cancer Institute. Image re-drawn for Omnigraphics by Alison DeKleine.*

The diaphragm (pronounced: dye-uh-fram), which separates the chest from the abdomen, plays a lead role in breathing. When we breathe out, the diaphragm moves upward, forcing the chest cavity to get smaller and pushing the gases in the lungs up and out of the nose and mouth.

When we breathe in, the diaphragm moves downward toward the abdomen, and the rib muscles pull the ribs upward and outward, enlarging the chest cavity and pulling air in through the nose or mouth. Air pressure in the chest cavity and lungs is reduced, and because gas flows from high pressure to low, air from the environment flows through the nose or mouth into the lungs.

As we exhale, the diaphragm moves upward and the chest wall muscles relax,

> ♣ **It's A Fact!!**
> ## Introduction To The Respiratory System
> When the respiratory system is mentioned, people generally think of breathing, but breathing is only one of the activities of the respiratory system. The body cells need a continuous supply of oxygen for the metabolic processes that are necessary to maintain life. The respiratory system works with the circulatory system to provide this oxygen and to remove the waste products of metabolism. It also helps to regulate pH of the blood.
>
> Source: SEER Training Module, Anatomy and Physiology, National Cancer Institute. Material undated. Accessed 6/19/2009: http://training.seer.cancer.gov/

causing the chest cavity to contract. Air pressure in the lungs rises, so air flows from the lungs and up and out of respiratory system through the nose or mouth.

Things That Can Go Wrong With The Lungs And Respiratory System

Many factors—including genetics, pollutants and irritants, and infectious diseases—can affect the health of your lungs and respiratory system and cause respiratory problems. Problems of the respiratory system that can affect people during their teen years include:

Asthma: Over 20 million people have asthma (pronounced: az-muh) in the United States, and it's the number-one reason that kids and teens chronically miss school. Asthma is a long-term, inflammatory lung disease that causes airways to tighten and narrow when a person with the condition comes into contact with irritants such as cigarette smoke, dust, or pet dander.

Bronchitis: Although bronchitis doesn't affect most teens, it can affect those who smoke. In bronchitis, the membranes lining the larger bronchial tubes become inflamed and an excessive amount of mucus is produced. The person with bronchitis develops a bad cough to get rid of the mucus.

Common Cold: Colds are caused by over 200 different viruses that cause inflammation in the upper respiratory tract. The common cold is the most common respiratory infection. Symptoms may include a mild fever, cough, headache, runny nose, sneezing, and sore throat.

Cough: A cough is a symptom of an illness, not an illness itself. There are many different types of cough and many different causes, ranging from not-so-serious to life threatening. Some of the more common causes affecting kids and teens are the common cold, asthma, sinusitis, seasonal allergies, and pneumonia.

Cystic Fibrosis (CF): CF is an inherited disease affecting the lungs. Cystic fibrosis causes mucus in the body to be abnormally thick and sticky. The mucus can clog the airways in the lungs and make a person more likely to get bacterial infections.

Pneumonia: Pneumonia is an inflammation of the lungs, which usually occurs because of infection with a bacteria or virus. Pneumonia causes fever, inflammation of lung tissue, and makes breathing difficult because the lungs have to work harder to transfer oxygen into the bloodstream and remove carbon dioxide from the blood. Common causes of pneumonia are influenza and infection with the bacterium *Streptococcus pneumoniae*.

☞ Remember!!

Although some respiratory diseases like asthma or cystic fibrosis can't be prevented, you can prevent many chronic lung and respiratory illnesses by avoiding smoking, staying away from pollutants and irritants, washing your hands often to avoid infection, and getting regular medical checkups.

Source: © 2007 Nemours Foundation.

Chapter 2

What Is Asthma?

There are many things that just seem to come naturally to some people. Maybe you know a girl who's a natural at sports—put her in a uniform and she's off and running. Some people are naturals at playing an instrument; it's like they were born knowing how to count in 4/4 time. Others are naturals at math; give them a test on theorems or equations and they're happy.

But some people have a problem with something that you'd think would come naturally to everyone: breathing. When a person has asthma, it can make breathing very difficult. And when it's hard to breathe, it can affect a person's game, that trumpet solo, and even the all-important geometry test.

What Is Asthma?

Asthma (pronounced: az-muh) is a lung condition that causes a person to have difficulty breathing. Asthma is a common condition: More than six million kids and teens have it.

Asthma affects a person's bronchial (pronounced: brahn-kee-ul) tubes, also known as airways. When a person breathes normally, air is taken in through the nose or mouth and then goes into the trachea (windpipe),

About This Chapter: Text in this chapter is from "Asthma," March 2007, reprinted with permission from www.kidshealth.org. Copyright © 2007 The Nemours Foundation. This information was provided by KidsHealth, one of the largest resources online for medically reviewed health information written for parents, kids, and teens. For more articles like this one, visit www.KidsHealth.org, or www.TeensHealth.org.

passing through the bronchial tubes, into the lungs, and finally back out again. But people with asthma have airways that are inflamed. This means that they swell and produce lots of thick mucus. They are also overly sensitive, or hyperreactive, to certain things, like exercise, dust, or cigarette smoke. This hyperreactivity causes the smooth muscle that surrounds the airways to tighten up. The combination of airway inflammation and muscle tightening narrows the airways and makes it difficult for air to move through.

In most people with asthma, the difficulty breathing happens periodically. When it does happen, it is known as an asthma flare-up, also known as an asthma attack, flare, episode, or exacerbation.

Asthma Flare-Ups

A person having an asthma flare-up may cough, wheeze (make a whistling sound while breathing), be short of breath, and feel an intense tightness in the chest. Many people with asthma compare a flare-up to the sensation of trying to breathe through a straw—it feels extremely hard to get air in and out of their lungs. An asthma flare-up can last for several hours or longer if a person doesn't use asthma medication. When an asthma flare-up is over, the person usually feels better.

Between flare-ups, a person's breathing can seem completely normal, or a person may continue to have some symptoms, such as coughing. Some people with asthma feel as if they are always short of breath. Other people with the condition may only cough at night or while exercising and they may never have a noticeable flare-up.

What Causes It?

No one knows exactly what causes asthma. It's thought to be a combination of environmental and genetic (hereditary) factors. A teen with asthma may have a parent or other close relative who has asthma or had it as a child. Teens who are overweight

♣ It's A Fact!!
Asthma isn't contagious, so you can't catch it from someone who has it.

may be more likely to have asthma, although a person doesn't have to be overweight to have it.

Asthma symptoms can be brought on by dozens of different things, and what causes asthma flare-ups in one person might not bother another at all. The things that set off asthma symptoms are called triggers. The following are some of the common triggers:

- **Allergens:** Some people with asthma find that allergens—certain substances that cause an allergic reaction in some people—can be a major trigger. Common allergens are dust mites (microscopic bugs that live in dust), molds, pollen, animal dander, and cockroaches.

- **Airborne Irritants And Pollutants:** Certain substances in the air, such as chalk dust or smoke, can trigger asthma because they irritate the airways. Cigarette smoke is a major cause of asthma symptoms, and not just for smokers—secondhand smoke can trigger asthma symptoms in people who are around smokers. Scented products such as perfumes, cosmetics, and cleaning solutions can trigger symptoms, as can strong odors from fresh paint or gasoline fumes. And some research studies have found that high levels of air pollutants such as ozone may irritate the sensitive tissues in the bronchial tubes and can possibly aggravate the symptoms of asthma in some people with the condition.

- **Exercise:** Some people have what's called exercise-induced asthma, which is triggered by physical activity. Although it can be especially frustrating, most cases of exercise-induced asthma can be treated so that people can still enjoy the sports they love.

- **Weather:** Cold or dry air can sometimes trigger asthma symptoms in certain people, as can extreme heat or humidity.

- **Respiratory Tract Infections:** Colds, flu, and other viral infections can trigger asthma in some people.

There are lots of other things that can trigger asthma symptoms in people with the condition. For example, a girl's asthma can get worse just before her period. And even laughing, crying, and yelling can sometimes cause the airways to tighten in sensitive lungs, triggering an asthma flare-up.

How Do Doctors Diagnose Asthma?

Many people with asthma are diagnosed with the condition when they're kids, but some don't find out that they have it until their teen years or even later. In diagnosing asthma, a doctor will ask about any concerns and symptoms you have, your past health, your family's health, any medications you're taking, any allergies you may have, and other issues. This is called the medical history.

The doctor will also perform a physical exam. He or she may recommend that you take some tests. Tests that doctors use to diagnose asthma include spirometry (pronounced: spye-rah-muh-tree) and peak flow meter tests, which involve blowing into devices that can measure how well your lungs are performing. Your doctor may also recommend allergy tests to see if allergies are causing your symptoms, or special exercise tests to see whether your asthma symptoms may be brought on by physical activity. Doctors occasionally use x-rays in diagnosing asthma, but these are usually only to rule out other possible problems.

Your family doctor may refer you to a specialist for allergy diagnosis and treatment. Doctors who specialize in the treatment of asthma include those who have been trained in the fields of allergy, immunology (how the immune system works), and pulmonology (conditions that affect the lungs).

How Is It Treated?

There's no cure for asthma, but the condition can usually be managed and flare-ups can be prevented. Asthma is treated in two ways: by avoiding potential triggers and with medication.

Teens who have asthma need to avoid the things that can cause their symptoms. Of course, some things that can cause symptoms can't be completely avoided (like catching a cold), but people can control their exposure to some triggers, such as pet dander, for example.

In the case of exercise-induced asthma, the trigger (physical activity) needs to be managed rather than avoided. Exercise can help a person stay healthier overall, and doctors can help athletes find treatments that allow them to participate in their sports.

Doctors treat every asthma case individually because the severity of each person's asthma and what triggers the symptoms are different. For this reason, doctors have a variety of treatment medications at their disposal. Most asthma medications are inhaled (which means that a person takes the medication by breathing it into the lungs), but asthma medications can also take the form of pills or liquids. They fall into two categories:

1.   Rescue medications that act quickly to halt asthma symptoms once they start. Some medications can be used as needed to stop asthma symptoms (such as wheezing, coughing, and shortness of breath) when a person first notices them. These medications act fast to stop the symptoms, but they're not long lasting. They are also known as "reliever," "quick-relief," or "fast-acting" medications.

2.   Controller medications to manage asthma and prevent symptoms from occurring in the first place. Many people with asthma need to take medication every day to control the condition overall. Controller medications (also called "preventive" or "maintenance" medications) work differently from rescue medications. They treat the problem of airway inflammation instead of the symptoms (coughing, wheezing, etc.) that it causes. Controller medications are slow acting and can take days or even weeks to begin working. Although you may not notice them working in the same way as rescue medications, regular use of controller medications should lessen your need for the rescue medications. Doctors also prescribe controller medications as a way to minimize any permanent lung changes that may be associated with having asthma.

Some people with asthma rely only on rescue medications; others use rescue medications together with controller medications to keep their asthma in check overall. Each person needs to work closely with a doctor to create an asthma action plan that's right for them.

Monitoring

In addition to avoiding triggers and treating symptoms, people with asthma usually need to monitor their condition to prevent flare-ups and help their doctors adjust medications if necessary. Two of the tools doctors give people to do this are:

☞ **Remember!!**
Dealing With Asthma

The best way to control asthma is prevention. Although medications can play an essential role in preventing flare-ups, environmental control is also very important. Here are some things you can do to help prevent coming into contact with the allergens or irritants that cause your asthma flare-ups:

- Keep your environment clear of potential allergens. For example, if dust is a trigger for you, vacuum (or remove) rugs and drapes where dust mites can hide. Placing pillows and mattresses in dust-proof covers can help. If pets trigger your symptoms, keep a pet-free household. If you can't part with Fido or Fluffy, keep certain rooms pet free and bathe your pet frequently to get rid of dander.

- Pay attention to the weather and take precautions when you know weather or air pollution conditions may affect you. You may need to stay indoors or limit your exercise to indoor activities.

- Don't smoke (or, if you're a smoker, quit). Smoking is always a bad idea for the lungs, but it's especially bad for someone who has asthma.

- Be smart about exercise. It's a great way to keep the body and mind healthy, so if you're prone to exercise-induced asthma flare-ups, talk to your doctor about how to manage your symptoms. If you get flare-ups during a game or workout, stop what you're doing until the flare-up has cleared or you've taken rescue medication. When the symptoms have gone, you can start exercising again.

Asthma doesn't have to prevent you from doing what you love! Sure, it takes a bit of work (and remembering) but if you follow your asthma action plan, take your medications properly, recognize your symptoms and triggers, and check in with your doctor regularly, you can do anything that other teens do. That includes any sports activity, even cross-country skiing, swimming, or playing basketball.

1. **Peak flow meter.** This handheld device measures how well a person can blow out air from the lungs. A peak flow meter reading that falls in the meter's green (or good) zone means the airways are open. A reading in the yellow zone means there's potential for an asthma flare-up. A reading in the red zone means the flare-up is serious and could mean that a person needs medication or treatment immediately—maybe even a trip to the doctor or emergency room. Teens who take daily medicine to control their asthma symptoms should use a peak flow meter at least one to two times a day and whenever they are having symptoms.

2. **Asthma diary.** Keeping a diary can also be an effective way to help prevent problems. A daily log of peak flow meter readings, times when symptoms occur, and when medications are taken can help a doctor develop the most appropriate treatment methods.

Chapter 3

Asthma Statistics

Asthma And Children

Asthma is a chronic inflammation of the airways with reversible episodes of obstruction, caused by an increased reaction of the airways to various stimuli. Asthma breathing problems usually happen in "episodes" or attacks but the inflammation underlying asthma is continuous.

Asthma is the most common chronic disorder in childhood, currently affecting an estimated 6.7 million children under 18 years; of which 3.8 million suffered from an asthma attack or episode in 2007.[1]

An asthma episode is a series of events that results in narrowed airways. These include: swelling of the lining, tightening of the muscle, and increased secretion of mucus in the airway. The narrowed airway is responsible for the difficulty in breathing with the familiar "wheeze."

Asthma is characterized by excessive sensitivity of the lungs to various stimuli. Triggers range from viral infections to allergies, to irritating gases and particles in the air. Each child reacts differently to the factors that may trigger asthma, including:

- respiratory infections, colds;

- allergic reactions to allergens such as pollen, mold, animal dander;

- feathers, dust, food, and cockroaches;

- exposure to cold air or sudden temperature change;

- cigarette smoke;

- excitement or stress;

- exercise.

Secondhand smoke can cause serious harm to children. An estimated 400,000 to one million asthmatic children have their condition worsened by exposure to secondhand smoke.[2]

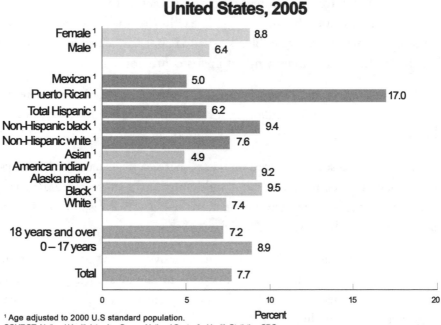

Percent of current asthma prevalence: United States, 2005

[1] Age adjusted to 2000 U.S standard population.
SOURCE: National Health Interview Survey, National Center for Health Statistics, CDC.

Figure 3.1. Percent of current asthma prevalence: United States, 2005. From Asthma Prevalence, Health Care Use and Mortality: United States, 2003– 2005. *National Center for Health Statistics, Centers for Disease Control and Prevention, October 2008.*

Asthma can be a life-threatening disease if not properly managed. In 2005, 3,884 deaths were attributed to asthma. However, deaths due to asthma are rare among children. The number of deaths increases with age. In 2005, 138 children under 15 died from asthma compared to 740 adults over 85.[3]

Asthma is the third leading cause of hospitalization among children under the age of 15. Approximately 32.7 percent of all asthma hospital discharges in 2006 were in those under 15, however only 20.1 percent of the U.S. population was less than 15 years old.[4]

In 2005, approximately 679,000 emergency room visits were due to asthma in those under 15.[5]

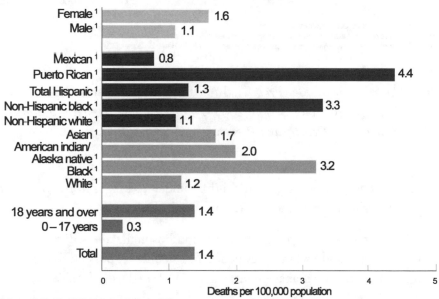

Number of asthma deaths per 100,000 population: United States, 2005

Category	Deaths per 100,000
Female[1]	1.6
Male[1]	1.1
Mexican[1]	0.8
Puerto Rican[1]	4.4
Total Hispanic[1]	1.3
Non-Hispanic black[1]	3.3
Non-Hispanic white[1]	1.1
Asian[1]	1.7
American indian/ Alaska native[1]	2.0
Black[1]	3.2
White[1]	1.2
18 years and over	1.4
0–17 years	0.3
Total	1.4

Deaths per 100,000 population

[1] Age adjusted to 2000 U.S standard population.
SOURCE: Mortality Component of the National Vital Statistics System, National Center for Health Statistics, CDC.

Figure 3.2. Number of asthma deaths per 100,000 population: United States, 2003. From Asthma Prevalence, Health Care Use and Mortality: United States, 2003–2005. *National Center for Health Statistics, Centers for Disease Control and Prevention, October 2008.*

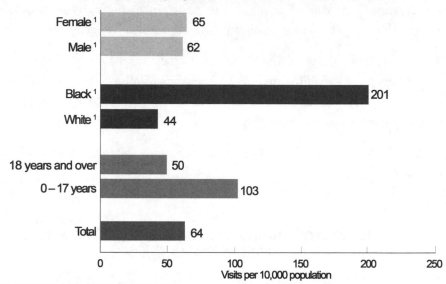

Number of asthma emergency department visits per 10,000 population: United States, 2004

Female [1] 65
Male [1] 62

Black [1] 201
White [1] 44

18 years and over 50
0–17 years 103

Total 64

Visits per 10,000 population

[1] Age adjusted to 2000 U.S standard population.
NOTE: Hispanic origin not available; estimates for race categories include both Hispanic and non-Hispanic persons.
SOURCE: National Hospital Ambulatory Medical Care Survey, National Center for Health Statistics, CDC.

Figure 3.3. Number of asthma emergency department visits per 10,000 population: United States, 2004. From Asthma Prevalence, Health Care Use and Mortality: United States, 2003–2005. *National Center for Health Statistics, Centers for Disease Control and Prevention, October 2008.*

Current asthma prevalence in children under 18 ranges from 5.7 percent in South Dakota and Idaho to 11.9 percent in Delaware.[6]

Within the last few years, mortality and hospitalizations due to asthma have decreased and asthma prevalence has stabilized, possibly indicating a better level of disease management, such as increased use of inhaled steroids.

Asthma medications help reduce underlying inflammation in the airways and relieve or prevent airway narrowing. Control of inflammation should lead to reduction in airway sensitivity and help prevent airway obstruction.

Two classes of medications have been used to treat asthma—anti-inflammatory agents and bronchodilators. Anti-inflammatory drugs interrupt the development of bronchial inflammation and have a preventive action. They may also modify or terminate ongoing inflammatory reactions in the airways. These agents include inhaled corticosteroids, cromolyn sodium, and other anti-inflammatory compounds. A new class of anti-inflammatory medications known as leukotriene modifiers, which work in a different way by blocking the activity of chemicals called leukotrienes that are involved in airway inflammation have recently come on the market.

Bronchodilators act principally to dilate the airways by relaxing bronchial smooth muscle. They include beta-adrenergic agonists, methylxanthines, and anticholinergics.

♣ It's A Fact!!
Who is at risk for asthma?

Asthma affects people of all ages, but it most often starts in childhood. In the United States, more than 22 million people are known to have asthma. Nearly six million of these people are children.

Young children who have frequent episodes of wheezing with respiratory infections, as well as certain other risk factors, are at the highest risk of developing asthma that continues beyond six years of age. These risk factors include having allergies, eczema (an allergic skin condition), or parents who have asthma.

Among children, more boys have asthma than girls. But among adults, more women have the disease than men. It's not clear whether or how sex and sex hormones play a role in causing asthma.

Most, but not all, people who have asthma have allergies.

Some people develop asthma because of exposure to certain chemical irritants or industrial dusts in the workplace. This is called occupational asthma.

Source: National Heart Lung and Blood Institute (www.nhlbi.nih.gov), September 2008.

In July of 2003, The Food and Drug Administration approved a new drug for patients with serious asthma. Xolair is the first in a new class of therapies that are bioengineered to target IgE (the antibody behind allergic asthma) in the treatment of allergic disease.[7]

Asthma is one of the leading causes of school absenteeism[9]; in 2003, asthma accounted for an estimated 12.8 million lost school days in children with an asthma attack in the previous year.[10]

> ♣ **It's A Fact!!**
>
> The annual direct health care cost of asthma is approximately $14.7 billion; indirect costs (e.g. lost productivity) add another $5 billion, for a total of $19.7 billion dollars. Prescription drugs represented the largest single direct cost, at $6.2 billion.[8]
>
> Source: © 2009 American Lung Association.

The American Lung Association funds a wide variety of asthma research. The American Lung Association-Asthma Clinical Research Centers (ACRC) network is an American Lung Association-sponsored research program seeking to develop large clinical trials that will provide useful information important to the direct care of people who have asthma. The network, with 18 clinical centers and a data coordinating center, is the largest of its kind. This work involves large numbers of subjects, making the focus of the network different from current federally funded and commercial research. Thus, the ACRC is playing a unique and important role in asthma research.

Table 3.1. Days Missed Due To Asthma Among Those Who Reported At Least One Asthma Attack In The Previous Year: United States, 2002–03

Days Missed	2002	2003
School days, children 5–17 years	14.7 million	12.8 million
Work days, currently employed adults 18 years and over	11.8 million	10.1 million

Source: From *Asthma Prevalence, Health Care Use and Mortality: United States, 2003–2005*, National Health Interview Survey, National Center for Health Statistics, Centers for Disease Control and Prevention, http://www.cdc.gov/nchs/, November 2006.

Currently the ACRC is conducting the Study of Acid Reflux and Childhood Asthma (SARCA) which will determine if poorly controlled asthma improves when acid reflux is treated with a certain class of drug, proton pump inhibitors. Acid reflux is frequent in people with poorly controlled asthma and can lead to asthma attacks. To find out if you qualify for participation, visit the ACRC section on the American Lung Association website, http://www.lungusa.org.

For more information on asthma, please review the Asthma Morbidity and Mortality Trend Report in the Data and Statistics section of the website at http://www.lungusa.org or call the American Lung Association at 1-800-LUNG-USA (1-800-586-4872).

Sources

1. Centers for Disease Control and Prevention: National Center for Health Statistics, National Health Interview Survey Raw Data, 2007. Analysis by the American Lung Association Research and Program Services Division using SPSS and SUDAAN software.

2. California Environmental Protection Agency: Respiratory Health Effect of Passive Smoking, June 2005.

3. Centers for Disease Control and Prevention. National Center for Health Statistics. Final Vital Statistics Report. Deaths: Final Data for 2005. April 24, 2008. Vol. 56, No. 10.

4. Centers for Disease Control and Prevention: National Center for Health Statistics, National Hospital Discharge Survey, 2006. Unpublished data provided upon special request to the NCHS.

5. Centers for Disease Control and Prevention: National Center for Health Statistics, National Hospital Ambulatory Medical Care Survey, 2005. Unpublished data provided upon special request to the NCHS.

6. Centers for Disease Control and Prevention: National Center for Health Statistics, National Survey of Children's Health through State and Local Area Integrated Telephone Survey, 2003. Analysis by the American Lung Association Research And Program Services Division using SPSS and SUDAAN software.

7. Lanier, B.Q., Corren, J., Lumry, W., Liu, J., Fowler-Taylor, A., Gupta, N. *Omalizumab Is Effective In the Long Term Control of Severe Allergic Asthma.* Annals of Allergy, Asthma, and Immunology, August 2003; Vol. 91: pp. 154–159.

8. National Heart, Lung and Blood Institute Chartbook, U.S. Department of Health and Human Services, National Institutes of Health, 2007.

9. Centers for Disease Control and Prevention. National Center for Chronic Disease Prevention and Health Promotion. Healthy Youth! Health Topics: Asthma. December 7, 2007. Available at http://www.cdc.gov/healthyyouth/asthma/index.htm. Accessed on December 20, 2007.

10. Centers for Disease Control and Prevention. National Center for Health Statistics. Asthma Prevalence, Health Care Use and Mortality: United States, 2003–05. January 2007. Available at: http://www.cdc.gov/nchs/products/pubs/pubd/hestats/ashtma03-05/asthma03-05.htm. Accessed on October 5, 2007.

Chapter 4

Asthma In Children And Young Adults

About Childhood Asthma

Asthma is the leading serious chronic illness of children in the United States. In 2006, an estimated 6.8 million children under age 18 (almost 1.2 million under age 5) currently had asthma, 4.1 million of which had an asthma attack, and many others have "hidden" or undiagnosed asthma.

Secondhand smoke exposure in both adults and children is a risk factor for new asthma cases. Recent studies have suggested that children of smokers are twice as likely to develop asthma as the children of nonsmokers, and that even apparently healthy babies born to women who smoked during pregnancy have abnormally narrowed airways, which may predispose them to asthma and other respiratory disorders. This research was extended by a recent study that reported a child's risk of being diagnosed with asthma by the age of seven increased 23 percent if their mother smoked even less than 10 cigarettes a day during pregnancy. The chance of developing asthma increased to 35 percent if the mother smoked more than 10 cigarettes a day while pregnant. Data from several studies show that prenatal maternal smoking is a risk factor for asthma onset in children, especially young children. While the mechanism is not clear, it may be due to slowed lung growth.

About This Chapter: Text in this chapter is from excerpted from "Childhood Asthma Overview," © 2009 American Lung Association. Reprinted with permission. For more information about the American Lung Association or to support the work it does, call 800-LUNGUSA (800-586-4872) or log on to www.LungUSA.org.

Outdoor air pollution also worsens existing asthma. Outdoor pollutants known to trigger asthma attacks include ozone, particulate matter, nitrogen dioxide, and sulfur dioxide.

What Are The Signs And Symptoms?

Common symptoms include coughing (constant or intermittent), wheezing or whistling sounds audible when a child exhales, and shortness of breath or rapid breathing.

Any child who has frequent coughing or respiratory infections (pneumonia or bronchitis) should be evaluated for asthma.

The child who coughs after running or crying may have asthma. Recurrent night cough is common, as asthma is often worse at night. Chest tightness and shortness of breath are other symptoms of asthma that may occur alone or in combination with any of the above symptoms. Since these symptoms can occur for reasons other than asthma, other respiratory diseases must always be considered.

In a young child the discomfort of chest tightness may lead to unexplained irritability. They may complain that their chest "hurts" or "feels funny." Infants who have trouble feeding or who grunt during suckling may have asthma.

☞ **Remember!!**

Any child who has frequent coughing or respiratory infections (pneumonia or bronchitis) should be evaluated for asthma.

What About Hidden Asthma?

Until rapid breathing, wheezing, and coughing become obvious, the condition of many children with asthma will go undetected. These children with asthma usually suffer some degree of airway obstruction, and unless it is brought under control the children may suffer respiratory illnesses more frequently than necessary.

Hidden asthma, however, can produce so few recognizable symptoms that even a health care provider might not be able to distinguish abnormal breath sounds with his or her stethoscope, but it may cause subtle problems such as limitation of physical activity. Pulmonary function testing usually reveals these cases of airway obstruction.

What Usually Triggers Asthma?

Exercise: Running can trigger an episode in over 80 percent of children with asthma. Bronchodilator medications used before exercise can prevent most of these episodes. With proper control of asthma, most children with asthma can participate fully in physical activities.

There might be exceptions, such as prolonged running, especially during cold weather, allergy season or illness from a "cold." Swimming seems to be the least asthma-provoking form of exercise. However, there have been recent concerns about excessively chlorinated pools precipitating asthma episodes.

Infections: Respiratory infections, including the flu, frequently trigger severe episodes of asthma. Research indicates that these infections are most frequently produced by viruses, rather than bacteria. Antibiotics are of no benefit for viral infections and thus may be of little value in an asthma episode. It is important for all children with asthma to get vaccinated for the flu each year. The American Lung Association's Asthma Clinical Research Centers have shown that the vaccine itself will not precipitate an attack.

Allergy: Many children with asthma have their symptoms triggered by allergies. Allergic children can suffer reactions to ordinarily harmless material (such as pollen, mold, food, or animals).

The allergens involved are common indoor inhalants such as dust mites, feathers, molds, pets, insects (especially roaches), outdoor inhalants (molds and pollens), or ingested foods (milk, soy, egg, etc.). Foods are much less frequent causes of asthma. These allergens may produce low-grade reactions which are of no obvious consequence; however, daily exposure to these allergens may result in a gradual worsening of asthma.

Irritants: Cigarette smoke, air pollution, strong odors, aerosol sprays and paint fumes are some of the substances which irritate the tissues of the lungs and upper airways. The reaction (cough, wheeze, phlegm, runny nose, watery eyes) produced by these irritants can be identical to those produced by allergens.

Cigarette smoke is a good example, because it is highly irritating and can trigger asthma. Most people are not allergic to cigarette smoke; that is, there is no known immunologic reaction. Nevertheless, this irritant can be more significant than any allergen.

Outdoor air pollution also worsens existing asthma. Outdoor pollutants known to trigger asthma attacks include ozone, particulate matter, nitrogen dioxide, and sulfur dioxide. Children are already at greater risk from outdoor air pollution than healthy adults: they have smaller air passages which are blocked easier, they breathe

> ✔ **Quick Tip**
>
> **Note:** Chronic sinusitis in childhood due to bacteria can be a very stubborn chronic trigger for asthma. Treatment for 10 days with antibiotics may not be effective. In these children, sinus x-rays are frequently required to diagnose the underlying condition.
>
> Antibiotic treatment for three to four weeks or longer may be required to completely eradicate these infections. Asthma may also be triggered by an ear infection or bronchitis, which would also require antibiotic therapy.

more rapidly, and are less likely to acknowledge breathing difficulties resulting from pollution and limit their exposure. For a child with asthma, these concerns are especially relevant.

Weather: Children with asthma have cited a number of climatic conditions as trigger factors. Many identify cold air as triggering asthma. Pulmonary function studies demonstrate that breathing cold air provokes asthma in most children with asthma.

Emotions: A common misbelief is that children with asthma have a major psychological problem that has caused the asthma. Emotional factors are not the cause of asthma, though emotional stress can infrequently trigger asthma.

A child's asthma might only be noticeable after crying, laughing, or yelling in response to an emotional situation. These normal "emotional" responses involve deep rapid breathing which in turn can trigger asthma, as it does after running.

Emotional stress itself (anxiety, frustration, anger) also can trigger asthma, but the asthmatic condition precedes the emotional stress. Therefore, a child's asthma is not "in his or her head," as many people believe.

Emotions are associated with asthma for another reason. Many children with asthma suffer from severe anxiety during an episode as a result of suffocation produced by asthma. The anxiety and panic can then produce rapid breathing or hyperventilation, which further triggers the asthma.

During an episode, anxiety and panic should be controlled as much as possible. The parent should remain calm, encourage the child to relax and breathe easily and give appropriate medications.

☞ Remember!!

Secondhand smoke can cause serious harm to children. An estimated 400,000 to one million asthmatic children have their condition worsened by exposure to secondhand smoke.

Irritants must be recognized and avoided. Cigarette smoking certainly should be avoided in the home of any child with asthma. It has been shown that when the parents of a child with asthma stop smoking, the child's asthma often improves.

Treatment should be aimed at controlling the asthma. When asthma is controlled, emotional stress will be reduced and other emotional factors can then be dealt with more effectively. Any chronic illness, especially if uncontrolled, can have associated secondary psychological problems. More severe psychological problems require a specialist to help the child and his or her family.

Source: Reprinted with permission. © 2009 American Lung Association.

Chapter 5
Asthma And Diverse Communities

Racial And Ethnic Differences

According to the Centers for Disease Control and Prevention, asthma prevalence increases with age, but health care use is highest among the youngest children. Boys have higher asthma prevalence and death rates compared with girls throughout childhood. Of additional concern is the fact that non-Hispanic black and Puerto Rican children have higher prevalence rates compared to non-Hispanic white children. Puerto Rican children have the highest prevalence of all groups, 140 percent higher than non-Hispanic White children, whereas Mexican children have low reported rates. Black children have higher mortality rates compared with white children. The disparity in asthma mortality between black and white children has increased in recent years. American Indian/Alaska Native children have current asthma prevalence rates 25 percent higher and black children 60 percent higher than white children. Asian American children have the lowest prevalence rates. While data for prevalence, health care use and mortality are major indicators of the impact of asthma on children, asthma symptoms that are unrecognized or

About This Chapter: Text in this chapter is from excerpted from "State of Lung Disease in Diverse Communities," © 2009 American Lung Association. Reprinted with permission. For more information about the American Lung Association or to support the work it does, call 800-LUNGUSA (800-586-4872) or log on to www.LungUSA.org.

not severe enough to warrant emergency care or hospitalization can still lower quality of life.

Concern has also been raised that asthma may be underdiagnosed, particularly among minority children who have more restricted access to high-quality health care. A recent study examined racial/ethnic differences among currently symptomatic children in acquiring an asthma diagnosis to determine if relative underdiagnosis among children of color exists. Among those reported to have wheezed in the past year, 83 percent of Puerto Rican, 71 percent of non-Hispanic black and 65 percent of Mexican American children were diagnosed with asthma compared with 57 percent of non-Hispanic white children. Using non-Hispanic white children as the reference group, the approximate adjusted relative risk for physician diagnosis of asthma-given wheezing in the past year was 1.43 for Puerto Rican, 1.22 for non-Hispanic black and 1.19 for Mexican American children. Minority children were reported to have more severe wheezing symptoms. Even after accounting for this increased severity, children in racial and ethnic minority groups were as likely or more likely to have a reported asthma diagnosis than non-Hispanic white children.

♣ **It's A Fact!!**

• African Americans have the highest asthma prevalence of any racial or ethnic group with the exception of Puerto Ricans. The current asthma prevalence rate in African Americans is 11.5 percent higher than that in non-Hispanic whites. The difference between races is significant.

• African Americans are hospitalized for asthma at more than three times the rate of whites.

• The asthma age-adjusted mortality rate in Hispanic females (1.4 per 100,000 population) was lower than African American females (3.4 per 100,000), and slightly higher than non-Hispanic white females (1.3 per 100,000).

• Mexican Americans have the lowest asthma mortality and prevalence rates compared to all racial and ethnic groups and subgroups.

• Data from some studies indicate that Asian Americans have lower rates of asthma than most racial and ethnic groups, including Native Hawaiians.

African Americans

African Americans have higher rates of asthma than any other group with the exception of Puerto Ricans. In 2004, the asthma prevalence rate in African Americans was 11.5 percent higher than among whites. The prevalence rate was also 81 percent higher in African Americans than in Hispanics, except Puerto Ricans. In 2004, an estimated 4.9 million African Americans had been diagnosed with asthma in their lifetime; 3.5 million of them currently have asthma and 2 million said they experienced an asthma attack in the past year. African Americans also have higher rates of asthma mortality. In 2003, African Americans were almost three times more likely to die from asthma than were whites (3.2 per 100,000 versus 1.3 per 100,000 respectively).

Several studies point to racial differences in health services for patients with asthma. In 2004, African Americans were three times more likely to be hospitalized for asthma than whites and five times more likely to seek care at an emergency room.

In 2003, the risk of hospitalization for adult and pediatric asthma was highest among non-Hispanic blacks. Data showed that blacks were 3.8 times more likely to be admitted for pediatric asthma and three times more likely to be admitted for adult asthma, as compared with non-Hispanic whites. Being non-Hispanic black appears to be associated, independently from low income and low education, with an increased risk of mortality from asthma.

A 1999 Cleveland Clinic Foundation study of managed care patients hospitalized for asthma found that African American patients made more asthma-related emergency department visits (45.2 percent) than white patients (22.4 percent) during the year after their initial hospitalization. During the same year, whites made more asthma-related visits to their primary care doctor (70.2 percent) and specialist visits (38.8 percent) than African Americans, 47.6 percent of whom visited a primary care doctor and 27 percent of whom visited a specialist. Regular care from a primary care physician or asthma specialist can help patients keep their asthma under control and help prevent emergency room visits associated with asthma attacks. The Ohio researchers noted in their study that education programs are needed for low-income African American patients to improve asthma health care.

☞ **Remember!!**

Although asthma is found in all populations, it occurs at especially high rates among communities of color, particularly inner-city African American and Hispanic populations. Scientists have different explanations for the high asthma rates among communities of color. Some believe that inner-city living and socioeconomic factors such as poverty, stress, and low access to proper health care may contribute to asthma among urban minorities. Others believe that genetic factors are the main cause.

Studies on both socioeconomic and genetic factors have yielded inconclusive results. For example, Harvard University researchers found that children under the age of 26 months who lived in areas with higher levels of violent crime were up to twice as likely to have physician-diagnosed asthma as those who lived in low-crime areas. Children under the age of 26 months living in areas with high levels of violent crime were also 40 percent more likely to have physician-diagnosed asthma than children over the age of two living in the same neighborhood.

Results from the National Institute of Allergy and Infectious Diseases (NIAID) National Cooperative Inner-City Asthma Study suggested that there was a link between exposure to cockroaches and episodes of asthma. The NIAID researchers found that children who were both allergic and exposed to higher cockroach allergen levels were hospitalized for their asthma 3.3 times more often than allergic children who were not exposed to high levels of cockroach allergens.

A possible explanation for this disparity may be genetic differences between races. A study conducted by the National Heart Lung and Blood Institute identified several genes for asthma and for responsiveness to allergens, some of which may be more common among African Americans.

Hispanics And Latinos

In 2004, over 3.4 million Hispanic Americans had been diagnosed with asthma in their lifetime. Over 2.1 million Hispanic Americans reported that they currently have asthma and 1.2 million experienced an asthma attack in the past year. Asthma prevalence rates in Hispanics were significantly lower than rates in non-Hispanic blacks and non-Hispanic whites.

Studies suggest that Puerto Ricans may have higher asthma prevalence rates than non-Hispanic whites and any other Hispanic subgroup, while Mexican Americans may have the lowest rates of all groups. A study of more than 3,000 Hispanics in New York, found that Puerto Ricans reported a 13.2 percent asthma prevalence rate, compared to 5.3 percent among Dominicans and other Latinos, including Mexicans. The study noted that differences among Hispanic groups were not explained by location, household size, use of home remedies, education level, or by the country in which their education was completed.

♣ It's A Fact!!

Puerto Rican children have the highest asthma prevalence of all groups, 140 percent higher than non-Hispanic white children; whereas Mexican American children have low reported rates.

A recent study compared asthma-related clinical characteristics among 684 Mexican and Puerto Rican people with asthma recruited from San Francisco, New York City, Puerto Rico, and Mexico City. Researchers found that Puerto Ricans with asthma had lower lung function, higher risk of emergency department visits and longer asthma duration than Mexicans. The researchers also found that Puerto Ricans with asthma responded less to medications, such as albuterol, than Mexicans with asthma.

Just as in the African American community, Hispanics are also less likely than whites to receive adequate health care and preventive medicine. A recent article found that Hispanic children received fewer asthma medications than white children after adjusting for patient race, age, gender, insurance status, symptom severity and the number of primary care visits for asthma. The researchers reported that, overall, 94 percent of Hispanic children had not used preventive medications in the past year compared to 73 percent of white children.

Source: Reprinted with permission. © 2009 American Lung Association.

Chapter 6

Risk Factors For Developing Asthma

Risk Factors For Asthma: Why Me?

Anyone with asthma is likely to ask sooner or later, "why did this have to happen to me?" Answers to questions like this are never simple. However, many pieces of the puzzle are known, and they may help explain why people develop this disease.

Atopy: An Irritating Problem

The immune system is designed to protect your body against harmful bacteria, viruses, and poisons. However, in some people, the immune system will also react violently to some otherwise harmless substances. This problem is known as *atopy*, and can cause a number of bothersome conditions.

Nasal allergies, known as *allergic rhinitis*, are one of the most common forms of atopy. The nose is overly sensitive to substances in the air, and this leads to hormones in the nasal lining that increase mucous production, itching, and sneezing.

Food allergies are a similar type of problem, where cells lining the mouth, throat, stomach, or intestine react to substances taken in orally. This may cause swelling, vomiting, and in some cases, difficulty breathing or shock.

About This Chapter: This chapter begins with "Risk Factors for Asthma: 'Why Me?'" by David A. Cooke, MD, FACP, © 2009 Omnigraphics. Additional information about birth date and asthma is cited separately in the chapter.

Atopic dermatitis is another troublesome allergic disease. People with atopic dermatitis start developing rashes soon after birth, and continue to get them on and off for the rest of their lives. They tend to have very sensitive skin that is easily irritated by various substances.

Asthma is strongly linked to atopy and atopic diseases. Atopic sensitivity causes increased hormone release inside the airways leading into the lungs when allergens or other substances are inhaled. These hormones cause spasms in the muscles that control the size of the airway tubes (airway hypersensitivity). This makes it difficult to get air in and out of the lungs, and causes wheezing and shortness of breath.

Atopic diseases frequently occur together. For example, nearly everyone with asthma also has allergic rhinitis. Another common combination is allergic rhinitis, asthma, and a severe allergic reaction to aspirin. The more atopic conditions you have, the more likely you are to develop asthma. These relationships are almost certainly not coincidental, and are a sign that the same kinds of problems are causing all these conditions.

Genetics: You Can Pick Your Friends, But Not Your Family

A great deal of asthma appears to be inherited. The disease runs quite strongly in some families, and having a family member with asthma is a major risk factor for developing it yourself. It is believed that this is due to similarities in genes that control the immune system.

Your risk for asthma also appears to depend somewhat on your ethnic background. For example, African Americans are more likely to develop asthma than other groups. No one is sure why this is true. Theories include particular genes being more common in some parts of the world, as well as differences in exposures to pollution due to social conditions.

Gender: Boys Will Be Boys, And Girls Will Be Girls

Asthma does not practice gender equality. Boys are much more likely to develop asthma than girls, at least until around age 20. At that point, the risk is more equal, and later in life, asthma actually becomes more common in women. Why asthma follows this pattern is unknown, but the trends are quite clear.

✎ What's It Mean?

Atopy: When a person's immune system overreacts to harmless substances like pollen, mold, or foods.

Atopic Dermatitis: An unpleasant skin disease that usually appears soon after birth. Itchy rashes develop, and tend to recur throughout life. Usually, the rashes are on the inner elbows and the backs of the knees.

Airway Hyperreactivity: The tubes in the lungs that carry air are "twitchy," and any irritation causes them to squeeze tight. Air has a hard time getting in or out of the lungs.

Allergic Rhinitis: Allergies affecting the nose. This causes stuffy noses, drainage down the throat, and sneezing.

Source: © 2009 Omnigraphics.

Premature Birth: Not Ready For Prime Time

Premature birth is a risk factor for developing asthma. People who were born premature are significantly more likely to develop asthma. This risk is especially high in people who needed to be on a ventilator early in life, which is common among more premature babies. Having an abnormal environment early in life may lead to unusual sensitivity of the airways, which may become permanent.

Infections: Stop Bugging Me!

There seems to be a relationship between asthma and infections, but it's not a simple one. Many people develop asthma for the first time after a bad cold or pneumonia. It seems like these infections trigger the asthma, but the disease keeps going long after the sickness is over.

Scientists think that certain viruses may be particularly likely to cause asthma. However, just catching one of these infections isn't enough to give you asthma. It probably takes having asthma-prone genes, plus a viral infection, plus other factors, to give you asthma.

So, is living in a space suit the best way to keep from getting asthma? Interestingly, people who got more colds as young infants are less likely to get asthma than people who had their first colds later on. Some scientists believe getting exposed to infections early helps teach the developing immune system how to tell the difference between dangerous and harmless.

Air Pollution: Clearing the Air

Air pollution has a big impact on asthma. Dirty air makes asthma worse, but it also seems to help cause asthma in the first place. People who live in large cities are much more likely to develop asthma, and the dirtier the air, the higher the risk. It's not clear why air pollution makes you prone to asthma, but there's no doubt about the link.

In addition to generalized pollution, it is clear that some work-related exposures trigger asthma. Solvents, dusts, vapors, and various types of chemicals are common culprits. This disorder is known as occupational asthma. People with occupational asthma may notice that their symptoms worsen when they go to work or over the course of a work day. Often, they will improve greatly over weekends and vacations, and worsen again when they return to work. Avoiding the responsible substance is key to treatment.

Smoking: A Dirty Habit

It shouldn't come as a surprise that smoking increases your risk for asthma. Tobacco smoke contains several hundred chemicals, as well as hot gases and pieces of soot. These have a variety of irritating effects on the airways, and may cause airway hyperreactivity even in people who don't have atopy. Being a current smoker roughly quadruples the risk of asthma, and smoking may cause childhood asthma to recur, sometimes after years of having no symptoms.

Unfortunately, tobacco affects the risk of asthma even in people who aren't smokers. Exposure to second-hand smoke (smoke from other people's cigarettes nearby) doubles the risk of developing asthma symptoms.

♣ It's A Fact!!
Many causes of asthma can't be changed, but avoiding tobacco smoke is a major risk factor that you can control.

Source: © 2009 Omnigraphics.

☞ **Remember!!**
So, What Can I Do?

Unfortunately, nearly all of the risk factors for asthma are not things you can control or treat. However, they may help explain why you may have developed the problem. In the future, the known risk factors may help to point to new ways to treat the disease.

Source: © 2009 Omnigraphics.

Even more significantly, smoking during pregnancy appears to be a big risk factor for developing asthma. Women who smoke during pregnancy are much more likely to have children who develop asthma. It is believed that the poisonous effects of tobacco smoke cause permanent damage and abnormalities of fetal lungs.

Obesity: A Weighty Topic

Your weight affects your risk for asthma. It appears that fatter people are at higher risk for asthma than thinner ones. Some studies suggest that losing weight may improve asthma symptoms as well. No one knows why weight affects asthma, and the relationship was discovered only recently.

Can Your Birth Date Increase Your Risk For Asthma?

Originally published as "Children's Birth Date Can Increase Their Risk for Asthma," written by Dr. Fred Little for The HealthCentral Network, Inc. and first published on HealthCentral's asthma website www.MyAsthmaCentral.com, November 24, 2008. Copyright © 2008 The HealthCentral Network, Inc. All Rights Reserved.

Will the time of year when a child is born affect asthma risk? In this section, we discuss some very recent research that has grabbed media attention: the effect of birth during the time of year on the development of asthma in infants. There has been a well-known association between viral infection

> ♣ It's A Fact!!
>
> ## Can Obesity Cause Asthma?
>
> I saw a patient two weeks ago with asthma who asked me an important question: "Is my obesity making my asthma worse?"
>
> I explained that while obesity definitely contributes to shortness of breath in asthmatics, and that asthma control improves with weight loss, we are not sure whether obesity directly causes asthma. And there are some scientists who believe that people who are obese are at greater risk for worse swelling and inflammation in the bronchi (windpipes), leading to more wheezing. I reviewed her asthma medications with her and spent a few minutes reviewing the importance of weight control on overall health as well as controlling asthma symptoms.
>
> Here's some more background information on the obesity-asthma connection. Obesity is defined by one's body mass index (BMI). BMI is calculated by dividing weight in kilograms by the square of height in meters.
>
> ### Body Mass Index
>
> An ideal BMI is between 20 and 25—for example, a 65 kg person (143 pounds) who is 5 foot 8 inches tall (1.73 meters) has a BMI of 22. A BMI of greater than 30 defines obesity; the percentage of Americans who are obese has increased to about 20 percent from 12 percent in the last twenty years.

(typically from cold viruses and related viruses) in infancy and the risk of developing asthma in childhood. Until now, we haven't known whether early viral infection contributes to the development of asthma or if young kids who will become asthmatic just get early viral infections more readily.

The current research suggests that viral infection in infancy (less than one year old) actually contributes to the development of asthma later in childhood.

Risks Of Developing Asthma In Infants

The study that was recently released looked at the time of year during which babies were born and the risk of developing asthma around ages three to five. They were curious if being born three to six months before the peak winter virus season had any relationship to developing bronchiolitis (an infection of the smaller breathing tubes in the lung) and asthma. As expected,

This trend has been accompanied by an increase in the percentage of Americans who have asthma, and scientists have looked for a link between the two. It is clear from this research that people who are obese have more asthma than those who are not.

There are several ways in which obesity may worsen the risk and severity of asthma: breathing mechanics (how easy or hard it is to get air in and out of our lungs) are altered; obese individuals may be more prone to inflammation in the lungs; and problems occur in dosing medicines accurately. There is also good evidence that weight loss (especially after weight reduction surgery) leads to much better control of asthma symptoms. Nevertheless, while obesity is associated with asthma, we do not know if, or how, obesity directly causes asthma.

Whether obesity causes asthma or not, it is directly associated with several other health problems, such as diabetes and high blood pressure. The BMI is easy to calculate—anyone with a BMI greater than 30 should look for ways to decrease this—whether they have asthma or not. Overall health and lung health are directly connected.

Source: Originally published as "Patient Encounter: Can Obesity Cause Asthma?" which was written by Dr. Fred Little for The HealthCentral Network, Inc. and first published on HealthCentral's asthma website www.MyAsthmaCentral.com, June 27, 2006. Copyright © 2006 The HealthCentral Network, Inc. All Rights Reserved.

they found that timing of birth in relation to the winter peak viral time (four months before, almost to the day) was related to a higher rate of bronchiolitis. This confirms prior research that shows that the peak risk age for infants to get bronchiolitis is about four months of age.

However, they also found that babies born four months before the peak viral time had a 30 percent higher risk of developing asthma in childhood than kids born at different times of the year. This is the key finding: if asthma was associated with getting more bronchiolitis, there would be more infections in the kids that ended up getting asthma but no relationship between timing of birth and getting asthma. This concept is a little hard to grasp but quite compelling. And the study was not small—the researchers studied 91,000 kids born over five years in Tennessee, so the conclusions are robust and backed by strong data.

We need to remember that asthma is a disorder in which heredity (genes—who your parents are) and environment interact. Asthma (and allergies) is more common in the children of parents who have asthma. It does tend to run in families. But there are many children of asthmatic parents who never get asthma. This could be due to chance (which genes are passed on obviously varies from child to child) and environment. A 'high risk' child may not develop asthma in an environment where there are few allergens, or may develop asthma symptoms after moving to a new city or house, for example. In this study, the investigators made sure that the effect they were seeing was not due to these other predictors of asthma. Using sophisticated statistical analyses, they were able to find that timing of birth during the year was at least as strong and perhaps a stronger factor in predicting the development of asthma in childhood.

What Can Be Done?

The results from the recent study are both interesting and add significantly to our knowledge about the development of asthma in children. However, we still have much to learn in order to be able to apply these findings into practice. The main lesson for children at risk of asthma (and for all kids, for that matter) is to limit the risk of getting bronchiolitis. Bronchiolitis is a respiratory viral infection, and like others, peaks in the winter months and is transmitted both by direct contact and from respiratory secretions. It is important to wash hands well when around other kids who may be sick and be vigilant when in common play areas where there are a lot of kids, especially during the "high season."

There isn't much to say about the 'obvious'—timing of pregnancy to avoid birth four months before the peak viral season during the winter. It seems that, with respect to timing, most pregnancies do not turn out as planned—either too quickly or too slowly! This is especially true with the changing demographics of the work force and couples starting families later in life. If one were so inclined to time a birth during a lower risk period of the year, a couple could start trying to get pregnant in late winter/early spring. With a few months leeway, a child would be born early the following year.

Timing pregnancy is like timing the market—it usually doesn't work. The decision to start or grow a family is big enough—timing that decision based on probabilities of developing asthma is not worth the worry.

Chapter 7

Types Of Asthma

Types And Causes Of Asthma

Asthma is a disease of the lung that affects the bronchial tubes or airways. The term "asthma" comes from the Greek, meaning "to breathe hard." Medical terminology defines the condition as *reversible obstructive airway disease* (ROAD). Unlike other conditions that obstruct the airways, such as cystic fibrosis, chronic bronchitis and emphysema, asthma does not affect sufferers all of the time.

The lungs are a network of airways or bronchial tubes. The bronchial tubes are made of muscles and a mucous membrane. In a healthy lung, air moves freely through the bronchial tubes.

When an asthmatic person has an asthma attack the membranes inside the bronchial tubes release mucus and become inflamed. The inflammation causes the muscles to contract and create spasms. These muscle spasms are responsible for wheezing. Wheezing is the sound that can be heard as the bronchial tubes constrict and air tries to escape.

Attacks can vary considerably in their severity and are sometimes relatively mild, but the condition is nevertheless a dangerous one. An asthma attack can easily spiral out of control at any time. This is particularly true for children.

About This Chapter: Text in this chapter is from "Types and Causes of Asthma," reprinted with permission from www.LungDiseaseFocus.com. © 2009 Morefocus Media, Inc.

♣ It's A Fact!!
New National Study Links Asthma To Allergies

Researchers at the National Institutes of Health (NIH) have found that more than 50 percent of the current asthma cases in the country can be attributed to allergies, with approximately 30 percent of those cases attributed to cat allergy.

"It has long been debated whether people who develop asthma have a genetic propensity to develop allergies, or atopy," said Darryl C. Zeldin, M.D., a senior investigator at the National Institute of Environmental Health Sciences (NIEHS). "This new research shows that 56.3 percent of asthma cases are attributed to atopy."

Atopy is a condition that results from gene-environment interactions and can be measured by a positive skin test to allergens (or allergy-causing substances in the environment).

The study, available online in the *Journal of Allergy and Clinical Immunology*, was conducted by researchers at the National Institute of Environmental Health Sciences (NIEHS) and the National Institute of Allergy and Infectious Diseases, both parts of the NIH. The data come from the Third National Health and Nutrition Examination Survey (NHANES III), a nationally representative sample of the population of the United States.

"Sensitization to cat appears to be a strong risk factor for asthma in this study," said Zeldin. Zeldin and his co-authors, however, point out that some research shows that exposure to cats, particularly early in life, may be a protective factor.

"We are not advocating parents get rid of pets, but if you suspect that you or your child might have cat allergies or get asthmatic-like symptoms, you should consult with a physician about the best course of action for your family," added Zeldin.

The NIH researchers looked at skin test data for ten allergens. A positive skin test reaction to cat allergens accounted for 29.3 percent of the asthma cases, followed by the fungus *Alternaria* at 21.1 percent and white oak at 20.9 percent. "Each of 10 allergen-specific skin tests was strongly associated with asthma; however, after adjustment by a variety of subject characteristics and all the allergens, only skin tests to cat, *Alternaria* and white oak were independently and positively associated with asthma," said Peter Gergen, M.D., M.P.H, of NIAID's Division of Allergy, Immunology and Transplantation, a co-author on the paper.

Other allergens tested include: Ragweed, dust mites, Russian thistle, Bermuda grass, peanuts, perennial rye and german cockroach. Approximately 10,500 individuals participated in the skin testing. During these tests, skin was exposed to allergy-causing substances (allergens) and a positive test was determined by the size of the reaction on the skin.

"This study tells us that allergy is a major factor in asthma," Gergen said. "But this study also tells us is that there are many people who get asthma who don't have allergies. We need to do more research to understand what is causing the asthma that is not related to allergies."

"This study confirms that the environment plays a major role in the development of asthma," said Zeldin. "Given the complexity of this disease it won't be easy, but if we can prevent, block or reverse atopy, we could reduce a large proportion of asthma cases."

Reference

S.J. Arbes, P.J. Gergen, B. Vaughn, D.C. Zeldin. Asthma cases attributable to atopy: results from the Third National Health and Nutrition Examination Survey. *Journal of Allergy and Clinical Immunology* DOI:10.1016/j.jaci.2007.07.056 *(2007)*.

Source: From a *NIH News Release* dated September 27, 2007, National Institute of Allergy and Infectious Diseases.

New Classifications In Types Of Asthma

Although clear patterns do exist, the specific causes of asthma are far from straightforward. Until recently, the condition was divided into two clearly defined types of asthma: extrinsic (allergic) asthma and intrinsic (non-allergic) asthma. Today, asthma is divided into a number of different types:

- Allergic
- Non-allergic/intrinsic
- Exercise-induced
- Nocturnal
- Occupational
- Steroid-resistant

Allergic Asthma: Ninety percent of all asthma sufferers have allergic asthma. Allergic asthma is triggered by allergens—substances capable of causing an allergic reaction.

Causes Of Allergic Asthma: The causes of allergic asthma are wide ranging. At the top of the list are specific allergens, such as pet dander, pollen, and dust mites. People suffering specific allergen-induced asthma are usually very aware of the offending allergen and try to avoid it.

Pollutants, wood dust, smoke, irritants, chemicals, viral infections, bacteria, stress, emotion, and exercise are other frequently diagnosed causes.

Childhood Allergic Asthma: Most childhood asthma is considered an allergic type of asthma. Childhood asthma occurs more often in young boys than girls and out of all childhood illnesses accounts for the most missed days of school.

Research has concluded that maternal smoking can contribute to asthma or other impairment of infant lung function, even before the child is born. Continued exposure to cigarette smoking can irritate the respiratory tract and make infants and children particularly vulnerable to allergic asthma.

Intrinsic Asthma: Asthma is called "intrinsic" when allergies do not play a part. Intrinsic asthma is not likely to develop in children; its typical onset occurs after age 40. Possible causes of intrinsic asthma include respiratory irritants such as perfumes, cleaning agents, fumes, smoke and cold air, upper respiratory infections, and gastroesophageal reflux (GERD). Intrinsic asthma tends to be less responsive to treatment than allergic asthma.

Exercise-Induced Asthma: At least eleven percent of the non-asthmatic population experiences exercise-induced asthma. Many of these people have allergies or a family history of allergies.

Exercise-induced asthma can affect anyone at any age and may be attributed to the loss of heat and moisture in the lungs that occurs with strenuous exercise. Frequent coughing during exercise may be the only symptom of exercise-induced asthma. But in cold, dry conditions exercise-induced asthma symptoms can be more severe. Some common sense coupled with prophylactic medications for exercise-induced asthma can prevent the onset of asthmatic symptoms for sensitive individuals.

♣ It's A Fact!!
Non-Allergic Asthma

Non-allergic (intrinsic) asthma is triggered by factors not related to allergies. Like allergic asthma, non-allergic asthma is characterized by airway obstruction and inflammation that is at least partially reversible with medication, however symptoms in this type of asthma are **not** associated with an allergic reaction. Many of the symptoms of allergic and non-allergic asthma are the same (coughing, wheezing, shortness of breath or rapid breathing, and chest tightness), but non-allergic asthma is triggered by other factors such as anxiety, stress, exercise, cold air, dry air, hyperventilation, smoke, viruses or other irritants. In non-allergic asthma, the immune system is not involved in the reaction.

Source: From "Non-Allergic Asthma," © Asthma and Allergy Foundation of America (www.aafa.org). All rights reserved. Reprinted with permission.

Nocturnal Asthma: Nocturnal, or sleep-related, asthma affects people when they are sleeping and, although termed "nocturnal" (belonging to the night), asthma symptoms can occur regardless of the time of day a person is sleeping. Symptoms of nocturnal asthma tend to be their worst between midnight and 4 a.m. Nocturnal asthma can be triggered by allergens in bedding or the bedroom, a decrease in room temperature, and gastroesophageal reflux (GERD), among other triggers. An estimated 75 percent of asthmatics are affected by nocturnal asthma.

Occupational Asthma: Occupational asthma occurs directly as a result of breathing chemical fumes, wood dust, or other irritants over long periods of time. An estimated 15 percent of asthmatics have occupational asthma.

Steroid-Resistant Asthma: In the case of asthma medications, especially steroids, more is not better. Overuse of asthma medications can lead to *status asthmaticus*, a severe asthma attack that doesn't respond to medication and may require mechanical ventilation to reverse. To prevent *status asthmaticus*, follow your doctor's directions and take medication only as prescribed.

Resources

Aetnasm InteliHealth—Diseases & Conditions. (nd). *Types of asthma.*

American Academy of Allergy, Asthma and Immunology. (nd). *Types of asthma.*

Laitinen, T., Polvi, A., Rydman, P., et al. (2004). Characterization of a common susceptibility locus for asthma-related traits. *Science 304*, 300-304.

National Jewish Medical and Research Center. (reviewed 2003). *What causes asthma?*

Neenan, J. M. (2000). *Even low steroid doses can be trouble.*

Schwarz, A., Lieh-Lai, M.W. (updated 2004). Status asthmaticus. *eMedicine.com.*

Chapter 8

Exercise-Induced Asthma

Everyone needs to exercise, even people with asthma. A strong healthy body is one of your best defenses against disease. But some people with asthma have "exercise-induced asthma" (EIA). But with proper medical prevention and management you should be able to walk, climb stairs, run, and participate in activities, sports and exercise without experiencing symptoms. You don't have to let EIA keep you from leading an active life or from achieving your athletic dreams.

What is exercise-induced asthma?

Exercise is a common cause of asthma symptoms. This is usually called exercise-induced asthma (EIA) or exercise-induced bronchospasm (EIB). It is estimated that 80 to 90 percent of all individuals who have allergic asthma will experience symptoms of EIA with vigorous exercise or activity. For teenagers and young adults this is often the most common cause of asthma symptoms. Fortunately with better medications, monitoring, and management you can participate in physical activity and sports and achieve your highest performance level.

What are the symptoms of EIA?

Symptoms of exercised-induced asthma include coughing, wheezing, chest tightness, and shortness of breath. Coughing is the most common symptom of EIA and may be the only symptom you have. The symptoms of EIA may begin during exercise and will usually be worse five to 10 minutes after stopping exercise. Symptoms most often resolve in another 20 to 30 minutes and can range from mild to severe. Occasionally some individuals will experience "late phase" symptoms four to twelve hours after stopping exercise. Late-phase symptoms are frequently less severe and can take up to 24 hours to go away.

What causes EIA?

When you exercise you breathe faster due to the increased oxygen demands of your body. Usually during exercise you inhale through your mouth, causing the air to be dryer and cooler than when you breathe through your nasal passages. This decrease in warmth and humidity are both causes of bronchospasm. Exercise that exposes you to cold air such as skiing or ice hockey is therefore more likely to cause symptoms than exercise involving warm and humid air such as swimming. Pollution levels, high pollen counts and exposure to other irritants such as smoke and strong fumes can also make EIA symptoms worse. A recent cold or asthma episode can cause you to have more difficulty exercising.

How is EIA diagnosed?

It is important to know the difference between being out of condition and having exercise-induced asthma. A well-conditioned person will usually only experience the symptoms of EIA with vigorous

> **♣ It's A Fact!!**
> Exercise that exposes you to cold air such as skiing or ice hockey is more likely to cause symptoms than exercise involving warm and humid air such as swimming.

activity or exercise. To make a diagnosis, your doctor will take a thorough history and may perform a series of tests. During these tests, which may include running or a treadmill test, your doctor will measure your lung functions using a spirometer before, during, and after exercise. Monitoring your peak flows before, during, and after exercise can also help you and your doctor detect narrowing of your airways. Then, using guidelines established by your doctor, you can help prevent asthma symptoms, participate in, and enjoy physical activity. Your doctor will also tell you what to do should a full-blown episode occur.

Treatment and management of EIA

With proper treatment and management people with EIA can participate safely and achieve their full potential. Proper management requires that you take steps to prevent symptoms and carefully monitor your respiratory status before, during, and after exercise. Taking medication prior to exercising is important in preventing EIA. Proper warm up for six to 10 minutes before periods of exercise or vigorous activity will usually help. Individuals who can tolerate continuous exercise with minimal symptoms may find that proper warm up may prevent the need for repeated medications.

What types of medications treat/prevent EIA?

There are three types of medications to prevent or treat the symptoms of EIA. Your health care provider can help you determine the best treatment program for you based on your asthma condition and the type of activity or exercise.

The first medication is a short-acting beta2-agonist, also called a bronchodilator. This medication can prevent symptoms and should be taken 10 to 15 minutes before exercise. It will help prevent symptoms for up to four hours. This same medication can also be used to treat and reverse the symptoms of EIA should they occur.

The second medication is a long-acting bronchodilator. It needs to be taken 30 to 60 minutes prior to activity and only once within a 12-hour period. Salmeterol can help prevent EIA symptoms for 10 to 12 hours. This medication should only be used to prevent symptoms and should never be used to relieve symptoms once they occur because it does not offer any quick relief.

The third type of medication is cromolyn or nedocromil. They also need to be taken 15 to 20 minutes prior to exercise. There is also some evidence that taking these medications will also help to prevent the late phase reaction of EIA that is experienced by some individuals. These medications also should only be used as a preventative measure because they do not relieve symptoms once they begin. Some individuals use one of these medications in combination with a short-acting bronchodilator.

If you have frequent symptoms with usual activity or exercise, talk to your doctor. An increase in your long-term control medications may help. Long term anti-inflammatory medications such as inhaled steroids, can reduce the frequency and severity of EIA.

Teachers and coaches should be informed if a child has exercise-induced asthma. They should be told that the child should be able to participate in activities, but that they may require medication prior to activity. Athletes should also disclose their medications and adhere to standards set by the U.S. Olympic Committee. Approved and prohibited medications can be obtained from the committee hotline (800) 233-0393.

What types of sports are best for people with EIA?

Activities that involve only short bursts of exercise or intermittent periods of activity are usually better tolerated. Such sports include walking, volleyball, basketball, and gymnastics or baseball. Swimming that involves breathing warm and moist air, is often well tolerated. Aerobic sports such as distance running, soccer, or basketball are more likely to cause symptoms. In addition cold air sports such as ice hockey or ice-skating may not be tolerated as well.

☞ Remember!!

It is important to consult with your health care provider prior to beginning any exercise program and to pace yourself. With effective management, people with EIA can perform and excel in a variety of sports. Many Olympic athletes and professional athletes with exercise-induced asthma have excelled in their sports, many winning Olympic gold medals.

Remember, with proper medical management you should be able to walk, climb stairs, run, and participate in activities, sports and exercise without experiencing symptoms. Do not let EIA keep you from leading an active life or from achieving your athletic dreams.

Chapter 9

Nocturnal Asthma

Nocturnal asthma. Many parents know all too well the coughing, choking, wheezing and congestion that can keep their children—and the rest of the family—awake at night.

"When my three-year-old's asthma acts up, it definitely disrupts his sleep and mine," says Allergy and Asthma Network Mothers of Asthmatics (AANMA) member Rachel Gerke. "I know it is bothering him when he is really restless at night, crying or moaning and hitting the sides of the bed when rolling. And when I go in to listen to him he is either breathing faster, usually from his belly, his chest not rising, or I hear a whistle at the end of his breaths."

Rachel's family is not alone. More than 20 million Americans are affected by nocturnal asthma—also called *nighttime* or *sleep-related* asthma. The condition has been reported in medical literature for centuries.

Allergy and Asthma Network Mothers of Asthmatics consulted sleep experts—including parents—for advice to help you and your family get a good night's sleep.

Why We're Losing Sleep

When you breathe in, the lungs transport oxygen into the bloodstream, where it's carried to the rest of the body. When you breathe out, they transport the waste product—carbon dioxide—out of the bloodstream. How well this process works varies throughout the day as part of the body's natural circadian rhythm—an internal clock that regulates body mechanics over a 24-hour period. Lungs work best during the day, with peak lung function at about 4 p.m. Several studies show that 12 hours later—around 4 a.m.—lung function is at its lowest. The fluctuation is usually less than 10 percent. However, people with asthma can have up to a 50 percent difference between daytime and nighttime lung function.

In addition to rhythmic fluctuations, other factors contribute to worsening asthma symptoms during sleep. According to Eli Meltzer, MD, of the Allergy and Asthma Medical Group and Research Center in San Diego, California, "These factors include changes in the degree of inflammation, the amount of allergen exposure and the responsiveness patients have to their medications. Not only do short-acting bronchodilators wear off while patients are asleep, their effect over the 4–6 hours of their activity is less at night than in the day. These conditions result in patients waking up short of breath because they need to take another dose."

Gastroesophageal reflux (often called *acid reflux* or *reflux*), a back-wash of stomach acid into the esophagus, is also a contributing factor to sleep disturbance. AANMA member Carol O'Leary found reflux to be the cause of her son's sleep problems. "After two and a half years of sleepless nights, my son's acid reflux was finally diagnosed and treated. An effective treatment plan helped our whole family start sleeping better."

Researchers aren't sure exactly how reflux and asthma interact, but they do see a connection—adult studies suggest as many as 75 percent of adults with asthma also have reflux. Reflux can set off asthma symptoms. Because reflux is more common when a person is lying down, people with asthma may have more difficulty during sleep.

Another sleep-related condition that can worsen nighttime asthma is sleep apnea. This sleep disorder causes repeated pauses in breathing throughout the night—a serious problem in itself, but also one that can set off or worsen asthma symptoms. A recent study by the Cincinnati Children's Hospital Medical Center showed that women with asthma are twice as likely to have symptoms of sleep apnea as women without asthma.

"Please don't rule out sleep apnea as a cause of poor sleep—even in children!" says AANMA member Laurie Soares. "My 10-year-old son has asthma and allergies. He snored, was a mouth breather at night, was tired a lot and had poor height and weight growth. His father has sleep apnea, so with all those factors present we had my son's tonsils and adenoids removed. Since then, he sleeps quietly, is gaining weight and reports that he now has dreams!"

Allergens—like pollen or mold that cause allergic reactions—can also play a role in sleep problems. Exposure to allergens during the day may set off a chain reaction in the immune system that produces symptoms hours later, as can allergens in the bedroom like dust mites or animal dander.

Studies show that postnasal drip and congestion from allergies can cause multiple nighttime "micro-arousals." These awakenings are so brief that the sleeper doesn't even remember them, but they affect alertness the following day.

The Next Day

The effects of nighttime asthma and allergy symptoms reach beyond the bedroom. Children with nighttime asthma miss more time from school—and their parents more time from work—than healthy children. School and work performance can suffer when the family can't sleep. Children whose rest is disturbed by asthma symptoms have a higher incidence of psychological problems and poor school performance. Studies show that these children score lower on memory and time-limited tests. The most obvious signs that asthma is disturbing someone's sleep are fatigue, irritability, and reduced alertness the following day. According to Dr. Meltzer, other signs to look for include morning headaches, depression, and impaired concentration.

Doctors use the term "allergic fatigue" to describe the tiredness and general lack of energy experienced by people with nasal allergies. This condition is often blamed on antihistamine medications, many of which cause sedation. But recent studies show that, in addition to other factors, poor sleep quality contributes to the exhaustion people with allergies may feel all day long.

Clean Sleep

Eliminating allergens and potential asthma triggers in the bedroom can make a big difference in your quality of sleep. Allergy testing, combined with your symptom history, will help your doctor determine which specific allergens are triggering your asthma or allergy symptoms. Then you can focus your efforts on eliminating exposure to those specific allergens.

AANMA member Rachel Clarke reports, "We were amazed at the huge difference in our children's quality of sleep once we removed our carpeting and installed wooden floors. It was expensive—but well worth it."

Jan Frey concurs. After finding out her son was allergic to dust mites and mold, she says, "We ripped out carpeting, removed drapes and stuffed animals and got rid of the clutter that collects dust. We allergy-proofed not only his bed but also his brother's bed in the same room and our bed. We were amazed at the immediate improvement. His nightly wheezing and asthma flare-ups cleared and he now sleeps more deeply and soundly."

Christine Noriega took a multi-step approach to helping her son get a good night's sleep. "My son's eczema would flare up and keep him scratching all night and his asthma would get worse. First, we found out he had food allergies and eliminated those foods. This helped calm his eczema. We also found he was allergic to dust mites. We put dust mite covers on his mattress and pillows, wash his bedding frequently in **hot** water and put a HEPA filter in his room. When he comes in after playing outdoors, we get him into the bath right away to get rid of the pollen and other allergens. Then we rub Vaseline all over his body and put on cotton pajamas. This helps his eczema. All of these steps are helping calm his asthma and he's finally getting a good night's sleep."

If cleaning up the bedroom isn't enough to curb allergy symptoms, work with an allergist on treatment options, including immunotherapy (allergy shots), oral and nasal antihistamines, and nasal corticosteroids. Children 12 and older can also be tested to see if they qualify for a medication that reduces the number of antibodies responsible for allergic reactions.

✔ **Quick Tip**
Dealing With Dust Mites

Most children and even teenagers have well-loved stuffed animals that are full of dust mites. How do you get rid of those dust mites? You could turn the hot water heater up to 130° F on laundry day. Or you can make your child's stuffed animals "allergy friendly" by sticking them in the freezer overnight. This tip was first reported by AANMA president and founder Nancy Sander in "A Parent's Guide to Asthma" in 1989. After the deep freeze, wash and dry the stuffed animals to get rid of dust mite body parts and fecal pellets.

Ensuring Sleep

If you think you are having trouble sleeping due to asthma or allergies, monitor your symptoms, report any problems to your parents or doctor, and keep a sleep journal (this can be part of your daily symptom diary). Talk to your doctor about nighttime problems. "We need to control asthma both during the day and at night to maximize a patient's health-related quality of life," emphasizes Dr. Meltzer. If you notice excessive napping or drowsiness, school problems, hyperactivity or distractibility, ask your doctor to assess your nighttime symptoms. Talk about your sleep schedule, sleep environment, sleep-related symptoms, and behavioral issues. You should also carefully monitor your use of medication: Are you taking all doses on time? Adept at using a metered-dose inhaler or nebulizer? Check your inhaler technique at the next medical appointment and talk to the doctor about other medical conditions—like reflux and sleep apnea—that could be contributing to sleep problems.

Rachel Gerke says, "It has taken us all three years of his life, but we've finally started to get my son's asthma symptoms under control." Rachel makes regular appointments for her son with his allergist and asthma program coordinator. "He's had fewer asthma symptoms now that we fine-tuned his medication plan, put wood flooring in his room, removed all stuffed animals, started washing his bedding frequently and put dust mite-proof covers on his mattress and pillow cases. I also think that it made a difference to take the diaper wipes warmer out of his room—it gave off a scent from the wipes that I believe irritated his airways. It is all those little things that a lot of people don't think about doing in their sleeping environment that make a world of difference."

Asthma and allergies don't have to keep you from getting the sleep you need. Work with your medical care team to determine what's causing sleep problems and how you can solve them.

What's On Your Bed?

With all the mattress and pillow options available today, are some better than others for people with asthma and allergies? It depends on what's causing your sneezing and wheezing.

If you have dust mite allergy, the keys to a good night's sleep are using mattress and pillow encasements and monitoring humidity levels. Dust mites need two things to thrive: water (which they absorb from the air) and food (which they get from you in the form of dead skin cells). Keeping your bedroom's humidity below 50 percent will deprive dust mites of their water source, and a special cover over your mattress and pillow will deprive them of food. The mattress and pillow encasements will also protect you from allergens in mite body parts and poop.

☞ **Remember!!**

A word about mattress and pillow encasements: Old-style pillow and mattress encasements were made of plastic; they didn't allow air to flow through, so you'd end up sweaty, and they made a lot of noise when you rolled over. New encasements are made of tightly woven fabric that's soft and silent. Small pores allow air to pass through but are too small for dust mites and allergens to get through. When shopping for encasements, look for bound seams and a pore size (the amount of space between fabric threads) of 10 microns or less. Avoid coatings or lamination that can wear off in the wash.

New allergy-free and hypoallergenic pillows may not solve your slumber problems. According to the American Academy of Allergy, Asthma and Immunology, both synthetic pillows and feather pillows promote dust mite growth. And allergy to feathers is actually very rare. So select the pillow that's most comfortable for you and use a tightly woven pillow encasement.

Chapter 10

Occupational Asthma

What is occupational asthma?

Asthma is a respiratory disease. It creates narrowing of the air passages that results in difficult breathing, tightness of the chest, coughing, and breath-sounds such as wheezing.

Occupational asthma refers to asthma that is caused by breathing in specific agents in the workplace. An abnormal response of the body to the presence of an agent in the workplace causes occupational asthma.

The abnormal response, called "sensitization," develops after variable periods of workplace exposure to certain dusts, fumes, or vapors.

This sensitization may not show any symptoms of disease or it may be associated with skin rashes (urticaria), hay fever-like symptoms, or a combination of these symptoms.

How does asthma develop?

Asthma is triggered in several ways and most of them are not completely understood. For simplicity, we categorize them into two groups: allergic and non-allergic.

About This Chapter: Text in this chapter is from *OSH Answers: Asthma*, http://www.ccohs.ca/oshanswers/diseases/asthma.html, Canadian Centre for Occupational Health and Safety (CCOHS), © 2005. Reproduced with permission of CCOHS.

Allergic Asthma: Allergic asthma involves the body's immune system. This is a complex defense system that protects the body from harm caused by foreign substances or microbes. Among the most important elements of the defense mechanism are special proteins called *antibodies*. These are produced when the human body contacts an alien substance or microbe. Antibodies react with substances or microbes to destroy them. Antibodies are often very selective, acting only on one particular substance or type of microbe.

But antibodies can also respond in a wrong way and cause allergic disorders such as asthma. After a period of exposure to an industrial substance, either natural or synthetic, a worker may start producing too many of the antibodies called *immunoglobulin E* (IgE). These antibodies attach to specific cells in the lung in a process known as "sensitization."

> ☞ **Remember!!**
> Not all workers react with an asthmatic response when exposed to industrial agents. Asthma strikes only a fraction of workers. Asthmatic attacks can be controlled either by ending exposure to the agent responsible or by medical treatment.

When re-exposure occurs, the lung cells with attached IgE antibodies react with the substance. This reaction results in the release of chemicals such as leukotrienes that are made in the body. Leukotrienes provoke the contraction of some muscles in the airways. This causes the narrowing of air passages which is characteristic of asthma.

Non-Allergic Asthma: Following repeated exposure to an industrial chemical, substances such as leukotrienes are released in the lungs. Again, the leukotriene causes narrowing of air passages typical of asthma. The reasons for such release are still not clear because no antibody reaction seems to be involved.

Other Types Of Asthma: In certain circumstances, symptoms of asthma may develop suddenly (within 24 hours) following exposure to high airborne concentrations of respiratory irritants such as chlorine. This condition is known as reactive airways dysfunction syndrome (RADS). The symptoms may persist for months or years when the sensitized person is re-exposed to irritants. RADS is controversial because of its rarity and the lack of good information on how the lungs are affected and the range of substances which cause it.

How long does asthma take to develop?

There is no fixed period of time in which asthma can develop. Asthma as a disease may develop from a few weeks to many years after the initial exposure. Studies carried out on some platinum refinery workers show that in most cases asthma develops in six to 12 months. But it may occur within 10 days or be delayed for as long as 25 years.

Table 10.1. Causes Of Occupational Asthma: Grains, Flours, Plants And Gums

Occupation	Agent
Bakers, millers	Wheat
Chemists, coffee bean baggers and handlers, gardeners, millers, oil industry workers, farmers	Castor beans
Cigarette factory workers	Tobacco dust
Drug manufacturers, mold makers in sweet factories, printers	Gum acacia
Farmers, grain handlers	Grain dust
Gum manufacturers, sweet makers	Gum tragacanth
Strawberry growers	Strawberry pollen
Tea sifters and packers	Tea dust
Tobacco farmers	Tobacco leaf
Woolen industry workers	Wool

Analysis of the respiratory responses of sensitized workers has established three basic patterns of asthmatic attacks, as follows:

Immediate: Typically develops within minutes of exposure and is at its worst after approximately 20 minutes; recovery takes about two hours.

Late: Can occur in different forms. It usually starts several hours after exposure and is at its worst after about four to eight hours with recovery

Table 10.2. Causes Of Occupational Asthma: Animals, Insects, And Fungi

Occupation	Agent
Bird fanciers	Avian proteins
Cosmetic manufacturers	Carmine
Entomologists	Moths, butterflies
Feather pluckers	Feathers
Field contact workers	Crickets
Fish bait breeders	Bee moths
Flour mill workers, bakers, farm workers, grain handlers	Grain storage mites, Alternaria, aspergillus
Laboratory workers	Locusts, cockroaches, grain weevils, rats, mice, guinea pigs, rabbits
Mushroom cultivators	Mushroom spores
Oyster farmers	Hoya
Pea sorters	Mexican bean weevils
Pigeon breeders	Pigeons
Poultry workers	Chickens
Prawn processors	Prawns
Silkworm sericulturers	Silkworms
Zoological museum curators	Beetles

within 24 hours. However, it can start one hour after exposure with recovery in three to four hours. In some cases, it may start at night, with a tendency to recur at the same time for a few nights following a single exposure.

Dual Or Combined: Is the occurrence of both immediate and late types of asthma.

How common is asthma?

The frequency of occupational asthma is unknown, although various estimates are available. In Japan, 15 percent of asthma in males is believed to be occupational. In the United States, two percent of all cases of asthma are thought to be of occupational origin. The number of cases of occupational asthma varies from country to country and from industry to industry. About six percent of animal handlers develop asthma due to animal hair or dust. Between 10 and 45 percent of workers who process subtilisins, the "proteolytic enzymes" like *Bacillus subtilis* in the detergent industry develop asthma. However, preparations of the enzymes in granulated form, which is less readily inhaled, have reduced the likelihood of asthma. Approximately five percent of workers exposed to such chemicals as isocyanates and certain wood dusts develop asthma.

What factors increase the chances of developing asthma?

Some workplace conditions seem to increase the likelihood that workers will develop asthma, but their importance is not fully known. Factors such as the properties of the chemicals, and the amount and duration of exposure are obviously important. However, because only a fraction of exposed workers are affected, factors unique to individual workers can also be important. Such factors include the ability of some people to produce abnormal amounts of IgE antibodies. The contribution of cigarette smoking to asthma is not known. But smokers are more likely than nonsmokers to develop respiratory problems in general.

How does the doctor know if a worker has asthma?

Sufferers from occupational asthma experience attacks of difficult breathing, tightness of the chest, coughing, and breath sounds such as wheezing,

Table 10.3. Causes Of Occupational Asthma: Chemicals And Materials

Occupation	Agent
Aircraft fitters	Triethylenetetramine
Aluminum cable solderers	Aminoethylethanolamine
Aluminum pot room workers	Fluorine
Autobody workers	Acrylates (resins, glues, sealants, adhesives)
Brewery workers	Chloramine-T
Chemical plant workers, pulp mill workers	Chlorine
Dye weighers	Levafix brilliant yellow, drimarene brilliant yellow and blue, cibachrome brilliant scarlet
Electronics workers	Colophony
Epoxy resin manufacturers	Tetrachlorophthalic anhydride
Foundry mold makers	Furan-based resin binder systems
Fur dyers	Para-phenylenediamine
Hairdressers	Persulfate salts
Health care workers	Glutaraldehyde, latex
Laboratory workers, nurses, phenolic resin molders	Formalin/formaldehyde
Meat wrappers	Polyvinyl chloride vapor
Paint manufacturers, plastic molders, tool setters	Phthalic anhydride
Paint sprayers	Dimethylethanolamine
Photographic workers, shellac manufacturers	Ethylenediamine
Refrigeration industry workers	Chlorofluorocarbons (CFCs)
Solderers	Polyether alcohol, polypropylene glycol

which is associated with air-flow obstruction. Such symptoms should raise the suspicion of asthma. Typically these symptoms are worse on working days, often awakening the patient at night, and improving when the person is away from work. While off work, sufferers from occupational asthma may still have chest symptoms when exposed to airway irritants such as dusts, or fumes, or upon exercise. Itchy and watery eyes, sneezing, stuffy and runny nose, and skin rashes are other symptoms often associated with asthma.

Lung function tests and skin tests can help to confirm the disease. But some patients with occupational asthma may have normal lung function as well as negative skin tests.

Table 10.4. Causes Of Occupational Asthma: Isocyanates And Metals

Occupation	Agent
Boat builders, foam manufacturers, office workers, plastics factory workers, refrigerator manufacturers, toluene diisocyanate (TDI) manufacturers/users, printers, laminators, tinners, toy makers	Toluene diisocyanate
Boiler cleaners, gas turbine cleaners	Vanadium
Car sprayers	Hexamethylene diisocyanate
Cement workers	Potassium dichromate
Chrome platers, chrome polishers	Sodium bichromate, chromic acid, potassium chromate
Nickel platers	Nickel sulphate
Platinum chemists	Chloroplatinic acid
Platinum refiners	Platinum salts
Polyurethane foam manufacturers, printers, laminators	Diphenylmethane diisocyanate
Rubber workers	Naphthalene diisocyanate
Tungsten carbide grinders	Cobalt
Welders	Stainless steel fumes

Table 10.5. Causes Of Occupational Asthma: Drugs And Enzymes

Occupation	Agent
Ampicillin manufacturers	Phenylglycine acid chloride
Detergent manufacturers	Bacillus subtilis
Enzyme manufacturers	Fungal alpha-amylase
Food technologists, laboratory workers	Papain
Pharmacists	Gentian powder, flaviastase
Pharmaceutical workers	Methyldopa, salbutamol, dichloramine, piperazine dihydrochloride, spiramycin, penicillins, sulfathiazole, sulfonechloramides, chloramine-T, phosdrin, pancreatic extracts
Poultry workers	Amprolium hydrochloride
Process workers, plastic polymer production workers	Trypsin, bromelin

Table 10.6. Causes Of Occupational Asthma: Woods

Occupation	Agent
Carpenters, timber millers, woodworkers	Western red cedar, cedar of Lebanon, iroko, California redwood, ramin, African zebrawood
Sawmill workers, pattern makers	Mansonia, oak, mahogany, abiruana
Wood finishers	Cocabolla
Wood machinists	Kejaat

✔ Quick Tip
How can we prevent occupational asthma?

The best way to prevent occupational asthma is to replace dangerous substances with less harmful ones. Where this is not possible, exposure should be minimized through engineering controls such as ventilation and enclosures of processes.

Education of workers is also very important. Proper handling procedures, avoidance of spills and good housekeeping reduce the occurrence of occupational asthma

The diagnosis of work-related asthma needs to be confirmed objectively. This can be done by carrying out pulmonary function tests at work and off work. Specific inhalation challenges can demonstrate the occupational origin of asthma and may identify the agents responsible when the cause is uncertain. Specific inhalation challenge tests require breathing in small quantities of industrial agents that may induce an attack of asthma. But they are safe when performed by experienced physicians in specialized centers.

How can we control occupational asthma?

Although there are drugs that may control the symptoms of asthma, it is important to stop exposure. If the exposure to the causal agent is not stopped, treatment will be needed continuously and the breathing problems may become permanent. People may continue to suffer from occupational asthma even after removal from exposure. For example, a follow-up study of 75 patients with asthma caused by red cedar dust showed that only half the patients recovered. The remaining half continued to have asthmatic attacks for a period of one to nine years after the termination of exposure.

Dust masks and respirators can help to control workplace exposure. However, these protective devices, in order to be effective, must be carefully selected, properly fitted and well maintained. Preventing further exposure might involve a change of job. If a job change is not feasible, relocation to another area of the plant with no exposure may be essential.

What occupations are at risk for asthma?

Some of the occupations where asthma has been seen are listed in Tables 10.1 through 10.6. It should be noted that the lists of occupational substances and microbes which can cause asthma are not complete. New causes continue to be added. New materials and new processes introduce new exposures and create new risks.

Part Two

Diagnosing And Managing Asthma

Chapter 11

How To Tell If You Have Asthma

Have you, or someone you know, been diagnosed with asthma? If so, you probably have lots of questions.

You may wonder, for example, just what asthma is. The medical definition of asthma is simple, but the condition itself is quite complex.

Doctors define asthma as a "chronic inflammatory disease of the airway" that causes the following symptoms:

• Chronic (regular) cough

• Shortness of breath

• Wheezing

• A feeling of tightness in the chest

If you suspect you might have asthma, your doctor will evaluate your medical history and your family's and also perform lung-function tests. Additionally, he or she may prescribe medications that can conclusively determine whether or not you have asthma.

Being Diagnosed—Knowing For Sure If You've Got Asthma

Symptoms of asthma come and go; you may experience some of them and yet not know for certain whether you've got asthma or not. For example, you might experience trouble breathing with exercise or get more 'chest' infections than other people do.

Persistent cough is a common sign of lung disease. Coughing is a major feature of asthma, especially in children. If your infant or child coughs to the point of vomiting, discuss the possibility of asthma with your doctor. There are reasons other than asthma for a long-term cough, like whooping cough and postnasal drip.

It is important to talk to your doctor about all of your concerns and to ask lots of questions. Something that you may not think is relevant may be useful in pinpointing the problem.

Depending on your circumstances, your doctor will evaluate some or all of the following:

- your medical history;

- your family history;

- what your symptoms are, how frequently they occur, and whether they improve with medication;

- whether you have allergies;

- what your individual triggers are (that is, what things or situations tend to lead to your experiencing asthma symptoms);

- your lung function, using tests like peak flow monitoring and spirometry to determine how quickly you can expel air.

☞ Remember!!

Only a doctor can diagnose asthma. Conditions such as pneumonia, cystic fibrosis, heart disease, and chronic obstructive pulmonary disease (COPD) have to be ruled out before your doctor can be certain that you have asthma.

Associated Conditions

♣ It's A Fact!!

You are more likely to have asthma if you have a parent or close relative with allergies and/or asthma. Your chance of having asthma is also increased if you have a history of:

- wheezing, even though you did not have a cold;

- inflammation in the nose, called allergic rhinitis;

- eczema, an allergic skin condition.

Asthma And Allergies: Many people with asthma also have allergies, and your doctor may refer you to an allergist if you are experiencing asthma symptoms. However, just as not everyone who has allergies develops asthma, not everyone who has asthma has allergies. Researchers are still trying to determine the exact relationship between the two.

No one is born with an allergy, but you can have a genetic tendency to develop one. If both your parents have allergies, you will have a 75 percent chance of also developing them.

Asthma and allergies are related, but they are not the same thing. An allergy is a reaction to a substance that is usually harmless. These substances (allergens) can be inhaled, injected, swallowed, or touched. Being exposed to an allergen may cause irritation and swelling in specific areas of the body, such as the nose, eyes, lungs, and skin. Allergens like pollen, mold, animal dander and dust mites can make asthma symptoms worse by increasing the inflammation in the airways and making them more sensitive. The best way to find out if you are allergic to something is to have an allergy assessment done.

Rhinitis And Sinusitis: Rhinitis and sinusitis are different but related conditions, that often make asthma symptoms worse.

Rhinitis is when the lining of the nose becomes inflamed and it usually occurs after exposure to an aeroallergen such ragweed. Sinusitis is when the lining of the sinus cavities become inflamed and infected and this generally happens after a viral, bacterial or fungal infection.

If you have asthma and also develop rhinitis or sinusitis, your doctor may recommend nasal corticosteroid sprays or other treatments in addition to your regular asthma medication. By managing your sinusitis or rhinitis, your asthma will be better controlled.

Gastroesophageal Reflux Disease (GERD): GERD is short form for gastroesophageal reflux disease or acid reflux.

In most people, GERD is simply ordinary heartburn. Acid reflux can cause asthma symptoms, particularly coughing, when stomach acid travels up the esophagus and irritates the airways of the lungs.

If you do not respond to conventional asthma treatments, or if your asthma symptoms appear to be associated with heartburn, ask your doctor to have you checked for acid reflux.

☞ **Remember!!**
Talk To Your Doctor

As you have learned, asthma affects different people in different ways, and its symptoms can vary over time. That's why it's so important to work closely with your doctor or an asthma educator to determine the medications and management strategies that are right for you.

Chapter 12

How Your Doctor Diagnoses Asthma

How Is Asthma Diagnosed?

Your primary care doctor will diagnose asthma based on your medical history, a physical exam, and results from tests. He or she also will figure out what your level of asthma severity is—that is, whether it's intermittent, mild, moderate, or severe. Your severity level will determine what treatment you will start on.

Medical History

Your doctor may ask about your family history of asthma and allergies. He or she also may ask whether you have asthma symptoms, and when and how often they occur. Let your doctor know if your symptoms seem to happen only during certain times of the year or in certain places, or if they get worse at night.

Your doctor also may want to know what factors seem to set off your symptoms or worsen them. Your doctor may ask you about related health conditions that can interfere with asthma management. These conditions

About This Chapter: This chapter begins with information from "How Is Asthma Diagnosed?" *Diseases and Conditions Index,* National Heart Lung and Blood Institute (www.nhlbi.nih.gov), September 2008. Additional information about asthma classification is cited separately in the chapter.

include a runny nose, sinus infections, reflux disease, psychological stress, and sleep apnea.

Physical Exam

Your doctor will listen to your breathing and look for signs of asthma or allergies. These signs include wheezing, a runny nose or swollen nasal passages, and allergic skin conditions such as eczema.

Keep in mind that you can still have asthma even if you don't have these signs on the day that your doctor examines you.

Diagnostic Tests

Lung Function Test: Your doctor will use a test called spirometry (pronounced spi-ROM-eh-tre) to check how your lungs are working. This test measures how much air you can breathe in and out. It also measures how fast you can blow air out. Your doctor also may give you medicines and then test you again to see whether the results have improved.

✔ **Quick Tip**

You may need to see an asthma specialist if:

- you need special tests to be sure you have asthma;

- you've had a life-threatening asthma attack;

- you need more than one kind of medicine or higher doses of medicine to control your asthma, or if you have overall difficulty getting your asthma well controlled;

- you're thinking about getting allergy treatments.

Source: National Heart Lung and Blood Institute, 2008.

If the starting results are lower than normal and improve with the medicine, and if your medical history shows a pattern of asthma symptoms, your diagnosis will likely be asthma.

Other Tests: Your doctor may order other tests if he or she needs more information to make a diagnosis. Other tests may include:

- Allergy testing to find out which allergens affect you, if any.

- A test to measure how sensitive your airways are. This is called a bronchoprovocation test. Using spirometry, this test repeatedly measures your lung function during physical activity or after you receive increasing doses of cold air or a special chemical to breathe in.

- A test to show whether you have another disease with the same symptoms as asthma, such as reflux disease, vocal cord dysfunction, or sleep apnea.

- A chest x-ray or an EKG (electrocardiogram). These tests will help find out whether a foreign object or other disease may be causing your symptoms.

Diagnosing Asthma In Young Children

Most children who have asthma develop their first symptoms before five years of age. However, asthma in young children (aged 0 to five years) can be hard to diagnose. Sometimes it can be difficult to tell whether a child has asthma or another childhood condition because the symptoms of both conditions can be similar.

Also, many young children who have wheezing episodes when they get colds or respiratory infections don't go on to have asthma after they're six years old. These symptoms may be due to the fact that infants have smaller airways that can narrow even further when they get a cold or respiratory infection. The airways grow as a child grows older, so wheezing no longer occurs when the child gets a cold.

✎ What's It Mean?

Bronchoprovocation test: Using spirometry, this test repeatedly measures your lung function during physical activity or after you receive increasing doses of cold air or a special chemical to breathe in.

Eczema: A disease of the skin characterized by inflammation of the epidermis.

Sleep Apnea: A common disorder in which you have one or more pauses in breathing or shallow breaths while you sleep.

Spirometry: A test that measures how much air you can breathe in and out. It also measures how fast you can blow air out.

Source: National Heart Lung and Blood Institute, 2008.

> ### 👉 Remember!!
> ### Choosing An Asthma Doctor
>
> Pediatricians, general practitioners, internists, allergists and pulmonologists can all treat asthma and allergies.
>
> Allergists or immunologists are internists and pediatricians who have additional training in the immune system and special skills in evaluating and treating asthma and allergies.
>
> They become board certified when they pass an examination in the specialty area of allergy and immunology. Because allergists tend to see more allergic and asthmatic people than other kinds of doctors, they are more experienced in treating them.
>
> This is especially important because about 90 percent of children and 50 percent of adults with asthma have allergies that trigger asthma symptoms. Identifying and learning to control these allergies can be the key to better asthma control.
>
> Your primary care physician may refer you to an allergist to test you for allergies and to get your asthma under better control. Once your asthma and allergies are better controlled, you can expect to visit your allergist less often as he or she works with your primary care physician to keep your asthma in check.
>
> Source: From "Choosing an Asthma Doctor," © 2005 Asthma and Allergy Foundation of America (www.aafa.org). All rights reserved. Reprinted with permission.

A young child who has frequent wheezing with colds or respiratory infections is more likely to have asthma if:

- one or both parents have asthma;
- the child has signs of allergies, including the allergic skin condition eczema;
- the child has allergic reactions to pollens or other airborne allergens;
- the child wheezes even when he or she doesn't have a cold or other infection.

A lung function test along with a medical history and physical exam is the most certain way to diagnose asthma. However, this test is hard to do in children younger than five years. Thus, doctors must rely on children's medical histories, signs and symptoms, and physical exams to make a diagnosis. Doctors also may use a four to six week trial of asthma medicines to see how well a child responds.

Asthma Classification

From "Asthma Classification," © 2008 Family Allergy and Asthma (www.familyallergy.com). All rights reserved. Reprinted with permission.

Based on the results of your visit with an asthma specialist, your asthma will be classified in one of the following categories (based on National Heart Blood and Lung Institute guidelines):

Mild Intermittent Asthma

- Symptoms of cough, wheeze, chest tightness or difficulty breathing less than twice a week

- Flare-ups—brief, but intensity may vary

- Nighttime symptoms less than twice a month

- No symptoms between flare-ups

- Lung function test FEV1 [forced expiratory volume, one second] equal to or above 80 percent of normal values

- Peak flow less than 20 percent variability AM-to-AM or AM-to-PM, day-to-day

Mild Persistent Asthma

- Symptoms of cough, wheeze, chest tightness, or difficulty breathing three to six times a week

- Flare-ups-may affect activity level

- Nighttime symptoms three to four times a month

- Lung function test FEV1 equal to or above 80 percent of normal values

- Peak flow less than 20 to 30 percent variability

Moderate Persistent Asthma

- Symptoms of cough, wheeze, chest tightness or difficulty breathing daily

- Flare-ups-may affect activity level

- Nighttime symptoms five or more times a month

- Lung function test FEV1 above 60 percent but below 80 percent of normal values

- Peak flow more than 30 percent variability

Severe Persistent Asthma

- Symptoms of cough, wheeze, chest tightness or difficulty breathing continual

- Nighttime symptoms frequently

- Lung function test FEV1 less than or equal to 60 percent of normal values

- Peak flow more than 30 percent variability

The level of asthma severity will determine what types of medicine you will need to get your asthma under control.

Chapter 13

What Does A Pulmonologist Do?

Pulmonary Function Tests

Pulmonary function tests are a group of tests that measure how well the lungs take in and release air and how well they move oxygen into the blood.

How The Test Is Performed

In a spirometry test, you breathe into a mouthpiece that is connected to an instrument called a *spirometer*. The spirometer records the amount and the rate of air that you breathe in and out over a period of time.

For some of the test measurements, you can breathe normally and quietly. Other tests require forced inhalation or exhalation after a deep breath.

Lung volume measurement can be done in two ways:

• The most accurate way is to sit in a sealed, clear box that looks like a telephone booth (body plethysmograph) while breathing in and out into a mouthpiece. Changes in pressure inside the box help determine the lung volume.

About This Chapter: This chapter begins with text from "Pulmonary Function Tests: Spirometry," © 2009 A.D.A.M., Inc. Reprinted with permission. Additional information about pulmonary function tests is cited separately in the chapter.

✎ Weird Words

Pulmonologist: A pulmonologist is a doctor who specializes in the lungs and breathing. The pulmonologist understands the anatomy, physiology, and pathology of the lungs and is trained to diagnose and treat diseases of the lungs such as asthma, bronchitis, and emphysema.

—KW

- Lung volume can also be measured when you breathe nitrogen or helium gas through a tube for a certain period of time. The concentration of the gas in a chamber attached to the tube is measured to estimate the lung volume.

To measure diffusion capacity, you breathe a harmless gas for a very short time, often one breath. The concentration of the gas in the air you breathe out then is measured. The difference in the amount of gas inhaled and exhaled can help estimate how quickly gas can travel from the lungs into the blood.

♣ It's A Fact!!
Alternative Names:
PFTs; Spirometry; Spirogram; Lung function tests

Source: A.D.A.M. Inc.,
© 2009.

How To Prepare For The Test

Do not eat a heavy meal before the test. Do not smoke for four to six hours before the test. You'll get specific instructions if you need to stop using bronchodilators or inhaler medications. You may have to breathe in medication before the test.

How The Test Will Feel

Since the test involves some forced breathing and rapid breathing, you may have some temporary shortness of breath or light-headedness. You breathe through a tight-fitting mouthpiece, and you'll have nose clips.

Why The Test Is Performed

Spirometry measures airflow. By measuring how much air you exhale, and how quickly, spirometry can evaluate a broad range of lung diseases.

Lung volume measures the amount of air in the lungs without forcibly blowing out. Some lung diseases (such as emphysema and chronic bronchitis) can make the lungs contain too much air. Other lung diseases (such as fibrosis of the lungs and asbestosis) make the lungs scarred and smaller so that they contain too little air.

Testing the diffusion capacity (also called the DLCO) allows the doctor to estimate how well the lungs move oxygen from the air into the bloodstream.

Normal Results

Normal values are based on your age, height, ethnicity, and sex. Normal results are expressed as a percentage. A value is usually considered abnormal if it is less than 80 percent of your predicted value.

Normal value ranges may vary slightly among different laboratories. Talk to your doctor about the meaning of your specific test results.

What Abnormal Results Mean

Abnormal results usually mean that you may have some chest or lung disease.

Risks

The risk is minimal for most people. There is a small risk of collapsed lung in people with a certain type of lung disease. The test should not be given to a person who has experienced a recent heart attack, or who has certain other types of heart disease.

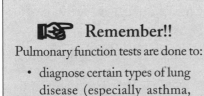

☞ Remember!!

Pulmonary function tests are done to:

- diagnose certain types of lung disease (especially asthma, bronchitis, and emphysema);

- find the cause of shortness of breath;

- measure whether exposure to contaminants at work affects lung function.

It also can be done to:

- assess the effect of medication;

- measure progress in disease treatment.

Source: A.D.A.M. Inc., © 2009.

Considerations

Your cooperation while performing the test is crucial in order to get accurate results. A poor seal around the mouthpiece of the spirometer can give poor results that can't be interpreted. Do not smoke before the test.

Pulmonary Function Tests (PFTs)

From "Pulmonary Function Tests (PFTs)" reprinted with permission from www.getasthmahelp.org, the website of the Asthma Initiative of Michigan, © 2009.

Pulmonary function tests (PFTs) are a series of different breathing tests led by a trained pulmonary function technologist, usually done at a hospital or clinic. There are national standards and guidelines that help make sure that everyone does and interprets pulmonary function tests in the same way. To learn about your lung health, your doctor may want you to have several pulmonary function tests done including spirometry, lung volumes, diffusing capacity, and arterial blood gases. Most of these breathing tests are done by blowing into a tube while sitting in a chair.

Before you have pulmonary function tests, you may get specific instructions on how to get ready for the tests, such as:

- wear loose clothing that will not restrict your ability to breathe deeply;

- avoid large meals prior to your test time which will make it more comfortable for you to breathe deeply;

✎ What's It Mean?

Spirometry: Spirometry measures many different volumes (how much) and flow rates (how fast the air moves). Some of the more common measurements done by spirometry include a test called forced vital capacity.

Forced Vital Capacity (FVC): Forced vital capacity measures the amount of air exhaled from full inspiration to full expiration (empty).

Diffusing Capacity (DLCO): Diffusing capacity of the lungs measures how well gases such as oxygen move from the lungs into the blood.

Source: © 2009 Asthma Initiative of Michigan.

- don't use your inhalers on the day of the test, if possible.

At your appointment, the equipment will be set up for you after being cleaned and disinfected, including a clean mouthpiece.

The technologist will tell you what to do before each test. Listen carefully and follow the coaching from the technologist. If you don't understand what to do, ask him or her to tell you in a different way.

Spirometry

Spirometry is a very common test to help you and your doctor understand your asthma better, and check how it is improving with treatment. The National Heart, Lung, and Blood Institute (NHLBI) guidelines recommend that all persons with asthma have spirometry done in the beginning of care, again as treatments are started, and at least every year for continuing care.

Spirometry measures how much air you can inhale (breathe in) and exhale (breathe out) as well as how fast you can exhale. For this test, you may be asked to breathe quickly, forcefully, or slowly. The test is always repeated at least three times and often more to be sure that the test is reliable.

Your doctor may order a bronchodilator to be given as part of spirometry. A bronchodilator is an inhaled medication that may dilate, or open up, your airways. Spirometry is often done before and after the bronchodilator to show any response to the medicine. Your response may help your doctor find out what kind and how much, if any, airway disease you may have, and whether you need medication to improve your breathing.

Forced Vital Capacity (FVC)

Forced vital capacity measures the amount of air exhaled from full inspiration to full expiration (empty). You will be asked to breathe in as deeply as you can and immediately blow out as hard and fast as you can until you feel you cannot blow any longer. With the help of a computer, the FVC effort will make a graph called a "flow volume curve" or "flow volume loop." This graph will look different for everyone. The measurements taken from this test are key in helping your doctor diagnose asthma.

Forced Expiratory Volume In The First Second (FEV1): FEV1 measures the amount of air you can forcefully blow out in the first second of the FVC. If this number is lower than what is considered normal, it may mean asthma. The ratio between your FEV1 and FVC, known as FEV1/FVC, can also help diagnose asthma. If your FEV1/FVC is lower than normal, it can mean asthma. It is normal for this number to go down somewhat with age.

Peak Expiratory Flow (PEF) Or Peak Flow (PF): Peak expiratory flow is the fastest flow rate reached at any time during a FVC. This depends a lot on your effort during the test.

Lung Volumes

The doctor may also order tests that measure your lung volumes. There are eight separate volumes of air that can be measured during the lung volumes test. The three most commonly used ways of measuring lung volumes are:

- **Nitrogen Washout:** Done by normal breathing of pure oxygen while exhaled gas is collected and analyzed.

- **Body Box:** Also known as plethysmography, is done while sitting in an enclosed clear chamber while asked to perform a series of very small panting breaths. This is the most accurate way to measure lung volumes.

- **Helium Dilution:** Done by normal breathing of gas mixture of helium and oxygen.

People with asthma may show changes in their lung volumes. This can help the doctor diagnose and treat asthma.

Diffusing Capacity (DLCO)

Diffusing capacity of the lungs measures how well gases such as oxygen move from the lungs into the blood. There are several ways to measure this, but the most common way is the ten second single breath-hold technique. Results of this test can tell your doctor about the amount of damage or abnormality that is present where the air and the blood meet. While this test does not specifically test for asthma, it may help your doctor to diagnose you correctly.

Arterial Blood Gases (ABGs)

This is a blood test that may be ordered with your PFTs to give your doctor even more information about your lung health. ABGs can show how well your lungs are getting oxygen into your blood and carbon dioxide out of your blood. For this test, a sample of blood is drawn from your artery, from your wrist or elbow area.

What We Can Learn From PFTs

A doctor will look over the results of your PFTs and see how you are doing by comparing them to predicted values normal for a person your age, size and sex. Height is important because taller people may have bigger lungs. There are many things that can change the results in PFTs. These include not only the health of your lungs but also the skill of the person testing you, your effort, differences in equipment, and differences in hospital or clinic procedures. A medical diagnosis is not likely to be made from PFTs alone.

Most lung diseases are labeled either as restrictive or obstructive. They are not the names of actual lung diseases, but the labels help group types of lung diseases together. Asthma is an obstructive disease, which means that it causes people to have trouble breathing out.

Words like mild, moderate, or severe may be used to describe how severe the problem is. Ask your doctor to explain the results so that you know what they mean for you.

☞ Remember!!

Keep in mind that quality of life is not found in the results of your PFTs. Each person is unlike any other, and many people live full lives with limited lung function. The key is to look for ways to keep or improve your quality of life, including exercise, breathing techniques, proper medications, equipment aids and social or emotional support.

Source: © 2009 Asthma Initiative of Michigan.

A PFT may be repeated as often as your doctor thinks it is needed. Lung problems can be checked for change by regular pulmonary tests. Check with your insurance company to see how often PFTs are covered for you—the NHLBI guidelines recommend them yearly for people with asthma.

Chapter 14

Should I See An Allergist?

Asthma and other allergic diseases are two of the most common health problems. Approximately 50 million Americans have asthma, hay fever or other allergy-related conditions.

Some allergy problems—such as a mild case of hay fever—may not need any treatment. Sometimes allergies can be controlled with the occasional use of an over-the-counter medication. However, sometimes allergies can interfere with day-to-day activities or decrease the quality of life. Allergies can even be life threatening.

The Allergist Treats Asthma And Allergies

An allergist is a physician who specializes in the diagnosis and treatment of asthma and other allergic diseases. The allergist is specially trained to identify the factors that trigger asthma or allergies. Allergists help people treat or prevent their allergy problems. After earning a medical degree, the allergist completes a three-year residency-training program in either internal medicine or pediatrics. Next the allergist completes two or three more years of study in the field of allergy and immunology. You can be certain that your doctor has met these requirements if he or she is certified by the American Board of Allergy and Immunology.

What Is An Allergy?

One of the marvels of the human body is that it can defend itself against harmful invaders such as viruses or bacteria. But sometimes the defenses are too aggressive and harmless substances such as dust, molds, or pollen are mistakenly identified as dangerous. The immune system then rallies its defenses, which include several chemicals to attack and destroy the supposed enemy. In the process, some unpleasant and, in extreme cases, life-threatening symptoms may be experienced in the allergy-prone individual.

The Cause Of Allergic Reactions

There are hundreds of ordinary substances that can trigger allergic reactions. Among the most common are plant pollens, molds, household dust (dust mites), cockroaches, pets, industrial chemicals, foods, medicines, feathers, and insect stings. These triggers are called "allergens."

Types Of Allergy Problems

An allergic reaction may occur anywhere in the body but usually appears in the nose, eyes, lungs, lining of the stomach, sinuses, throat, and skin. These are places where special immune system cells are stationed to fight off invaders that are inhaled, swallowed or come in contact with the skin.

♣ It's A Fact!!
Who develops asthma or allergies?

Asthma and allergies can affect anyone, regardless of age, gender, race or socioeconomic factors. While it's true that asthma and allergies are more common in children, they can occur for the first time at any age. Sometimes allergy symptoms start in childhood, disappear for many years and then start up again during adult life.

Although the exact genetic factors are not yet understood, there is a hereditary tendency to asthma and allergies. In susceptible people, factors such as hormones, stress, smoke, perfume, or other environmental irritants also may play a role.

Allergic Rhinitis (Hay Fever): Allergic rhinitis is a general term used to describe the allergic reactions that take place in the nose. Symptoms may include sneezing, congestion, runny nose, and itching of the nose, the eyes and/or the roof of the mouth. When this problem is triggered by pollens or outdoor molds, during the spring, summer or fall, the condition is often called "hay fever." When the problem is year-round, it might be caused by exposure to house dust mites, household pets, indoor molds, or allergens at school or in the workplace.

Asthma: Asthma symptoms occur when airway muscle spasms block the flow of air to the lungs and/or the linings of the bronchial tubes become inflamed. Excess mucus may clog the airways. An asthma attack is characterized by labored or restricted breathing, a tight feeling in the chest, coughing, and/or wheezing. Sometimes a chronic cough is the only symptom. Asthma trouble can cause only mild discomfort or it can cause life-threatening attacks in which breathing stops altogether.

Contact Dermatitis/Skin Allergies: Contact dermatitis, eczema, and hives are skin conditions that can be caused by allergens and other irritants. Often the reaction may take hours or days to develop, as in the case of poison ivy. The most common allergic causes of rashes are medicines, insect stings, foods, animals, and chemicals used at home or work. Allergies may be aggravated by emotional stress.

Anaphylaxis: Anaphylaxis is a rare, potentially fatal allergic reaction that affects many parts of the body at the same time. The trigger may be an insect sting, a food (such as peanuts), or a medication. Symptoms may include:

- vomiting or diarrhea;
- a dangerous drop in blood pressure;
- redness of the skin and/or hives;
- difficulty breathing;
- swelling of the throat and/or tongue;
- loss of consciousness.

Frequently these symptoms start without warning and get worse rapidly. At the first sign of an anaphylactic reaction, the affected person must go immediately to the closest Emergency Room or call 911.

When To See An Allergist

Often, the symptoms of asthma or allergies develop gradually over time.

Allergy sufferers may become used to frequent symptoms such as sneezing, nasal congestion, or wheezing. With the help of an allergist, these symptoms usually can be prevented or controlled with major improvement in quality of life.

Effectively controlling asthma and allergies requires planning, skill, and patience. The allergist, with his or her specialized training, can develop a treatment plan for your individual condition. The goal will be to enable you to lead a life that is as normal and symptom-free as possible.

✔ Quick Tip

You should see an allergist if:

- your allergies are causing symptoms such as chronic sinus infections, nasal congestion or difficulty breathing;

- you experience hay fever or other allergy symptoms several months out of the year;

- antihistamines and over-the-counter medications do not control your allergy symptoms or create unacceptable side effects, such as drowsiness;

- your asthma or allergies are interfering with your ability to carry on day-to-day activities;

- your asthma or allergies decrease the quality of your life;

- you are experiencing warning signs of serious asthma such as:

  - you sometimes have to struggle to catch your breath

  - you often wheeze or cough, especially at night or after exercise

  - you are frequently short of breath or feel tightness in your chest

  - you have previously been diagnosed with asthma, and you have frequent asthma attacks even though you are taking asthma medication.

A visit to the allergist might include:

Allergy Testing: The allergist will usually perform tests to determine what allergens are involved.

Prevention Education: The most effective approach to treating asthma or allergies is to avoid the factors that trigger the condition in the first place. Even when it is not possible to completely avoid allergens, an allergist can help you decrease exposure to allergens.

Medication Prescriptions: A number of new and effective medications are available to treat both asthma and allergies.

Immunotherapy (Allergy Shots): In this treatment, patients are given injections every week or two of some or all of the allergens that cause their allergy problems. Gradually the injections get stronger and stronger. In most cases, the allergy problems get less and less over time.

Chapter 15

Allergy Testing

Allergy Testing For Children

What is an allergy?

An allergy is the body's immune system response to specific elements in the environment. Children with allergies react to certain substances in their everyday environment, which usually don't cause reactions in other children.

About 20 percent of Americans—one in every five adults and children—have allergies, including allergic asthma. About 80 percent of children with asthma have allergies. Food allergies occur in eight percent of children younger than age six.

How do allergies affect children and how do they get them?

Children seem to be more vulnerable to allergies than adults. Allergies to food, house dust mites, animal dander, and pollen are most common. These allergies show up as allergic rhinitis (hay fever), asthma, and atopic dermatitis (eczema). Also, frequent ear infections may be related to allergy.

If both parents have allergies, their (biological) child has a 75 percent chance of having allergies. If one parent is allergic, or if relatives on one side of the family have allergies, then the child has about a 50 percent chance of developing allergies.

There is some evidence that breast-feeding helps prevent children from developing food allergies and eczema.

What are signs or symptoms of allergy in a child?

Symptoms develop as the body releases special antibodies called IgE (immunoglobin E), which are the key players in allergic reaction. These special antibodies can trigger the release of chemicals that can cause the physical symptoms and changes associated with allergies such as:

- hives;

- runny nose;

- itching or swelling of the lips, tongue, or throat;

- upset stomach, cramps, bloating, or diarrhea;

- wheezing or difficulty breathing;

- anaphylactic shock—a life-threatening body reaction requiring emergency care.

What tests are generally used to diagnose allergies?

First, keep in mind that allergy tests are not the sole basis for diagnosing or treating an allergy. Health care providers make an allergy diagnosis based on several factors:

- History of the patient's experiences and family history of allergy/asthma

- Physical exam of the patient to detect signs of allergy

- Allergy testing for sensitivity to specific allergens

Allergy tests help your physician confirm allergies you may have. When an allergy test pinpoints a reaction to a specific allergen(s), your health care provider also can use this information in developing "immunotherapy"— allergy shots—specifically for you, if appropriate.

Skin Tests For Allergies: Skin prick tests are the most common tests for allergy. Small amounts of suspect allergy triggers are introduced through the skin of the arm or back by pricking or puncturing the skin with a needle or similar device. If you are allergic to a substance, you will see a raised, red itchy bump, also called a "wheal." Reactions usually appear within 15 minutes. This positive result indicates that the IgE antibody is present when you come in contact with the specific allergen. The size of the wheal is important: the bigger it is, the more sensitive you are to that particular substance. This test is the least time consuming and expensive. You may have to discontinue certain medications, especially antihistamines, several days prior to testing.

☞ **Remember!!**
Allergy Overview: Diagnosis

If you break out in hives when a bee stings you, or you sneeze every time you pet a cat, you know what some of your allergens are. But if the pattern is not so obvious, try keeping a record of when, where, and under what circumstances your reactions occur. This can be as easy as jotting down notes on a calendar. If the pattern still isn't clear, make an appointment with your doctor for help.

Doctors diagnose allergies in three steps:

1. **Personal and medical history.** Your doctor will ask you questions to get a complete understanding of your symptoms and their possible causes. Bring your notes to help jog your memory. Be ready to answer questions about your family history, the kinds of medicines you take, and your lifestyle at home, school, and work.

2. **Physical examination.** If your doctor suspects an allergy, he or she will pay special attention to your ears, eyes, nose, throat, chest, and skin during the physical examination. This exam may include a pulmonary function test to detect how well you exhale air from your lungs. You may also need an x-ray of your lungs or sinuses.

3. **Tests to determine your allergens.** Your doctor may do a skin test, patch test or blood test.

Source: From "Allergy Overview: Diagnosis," © 2005 Asthma and Allergy Foundation of America (www.aafa.org).

Blood Tests For Allergies: The RAST (radioallergosorbent test) and related blood tests use radioactive or enzyme markers to detect levels of IgE antibodies. These tests are useful when a skin test is difficult due to a widespread skin rash, anxiety about skin pricks, or if the patient has the potential for a sudden and severe allergic response to test allergens.

Skin tests and these blood tests are very comparable in their ability to diagnose sensitivity to specific allergens. Both kinds of tests are considered to be about 90 percent accurate.

Elimination Diet: An elimination diet is often used to help isolate sensitivity to specific foods. Your health care provider sets up a diet without foods that you suspect may affect you. Because milk, soybeans, eggs, wheat, peanuts, nuts, shellfish, and corn are the main culprits for more than 80 percent of people who have food allergies, these foods are usually not included in the starting diet.

You will stay on the prescribed diet for four to seven days. If the symptoms do not subside, additional foods are eliminated until the allergy symptoms stop. Once the symptoms disappear, new foods are added to the basic diet, one at a time, until symptoms reappear.

♣ It's A Fact!!

There are four kinds of skin tests: scratch, puncture, prick, and intradermal. Your allergist may use one or more skin tests to analyze your response to various substances. Keep in mind that you may see a false-positive or a false-negative skin test. Results often depend on how well the test is performed.

Skin prick, puncture, and intradermal tests may be difficult with young children afraid of needles. There is some possibility of a life-threatening anaphylactic response if a person is extremely sensitive to a substance. Your health care provider will be prepared to react swiftly to this kind of response.

Source: From "Allergy Testing for Children,"
© 2005 Asthma and Allergy Foundation of
America (www.aafa.org).

The chief drawback to an elimination diet is making sure you eat "pure" foods. Common food allergens are "hidden ingredients" in hundreds of packaged or processed foods. In order for an elimination diet to be successful, check ingredients for foods you eat. For a fussy or picky eater, an elimination diet can be difficult. Your health care provider can suggest helpful approaches.

Fasting is a radical way to identify food allergies. Although very effective for detecting problem foods, this kind of elimination diet is hard to do with children. Fasting is best done under medical supervision and often is used for "extreme" cases where a child is suspected to have allergies to many types of food.

Are there other allergy tests?

The tests described above are considered the most effective and usual way to help diagnose allergies to specific substances. You also may hear of other allergy tests. These tests may work, but as yet, they are unproven or not universally accepted allergy testing methods. If your health care provider suggests one of these tests, consider getting a second opinion about allergy testing:

- Cytotoxicity blood test
- Electroacupuncture biofeedback
- Urine autoinjection
- Skin titration
- Sublingual provocative testing
- Candidiasis allergy theory
- Basophil histamine release

What kind of doctor does allergy testing?

Allergy testing usually is done by an allergist. An allergist specializes in diagnosing and treating allergies. Some allergists specialize in treating children. To find a board-certified allergist or pediatric allergist near you, contact:

- American Academy of Allergy, Asthma & Immunology at (800) 822-ASMA or http://www.aaaai.org

- American College of Allergy, Asthma & Immunology at (800) 842-7777 or http://allergy.mcg.edu

✔ Quick Tip

**What can you do if
you have a positive allergy test?**

A positive allergy test helps your physician figure out the best treatment plan for you. The doctor may prescribe specific medicine for the allergy(s) and suggest ways to cut down or eliminate substances in your environment that can trigger an allergic response. Many allergies are mild to moderate. Most allergies are easily managed with the right treatment plan.

Source: From "Allergy Testing for Children," © 2005 Asthma and Allergy Foundation of America (www.aafa.org).

Chapter 16

What Is A Peak Flow Meter?

A peak flow meter is a portable, inexpensive, hand-held device used to measure how air flows from your lungs in one "fast blast." In other words, the meter measures your ability to push air out of your lungs.

Peak flow meters may be provided in two ranges to measure the air pushed out of your lungs. A low range peak flow meter is for small children, and a standard range meter is for older children, teenagers, and adults. An adult has much larger airways than a child and needs the larger range.

Who can benefit from using a peak flow meter?

Not all physicians use peak flow meters in their management of children and adults with asthma. Many health care providers believe a peak flow meter may be of most help for people with moderate and severe asthma. If your asthma is mild or you do not use daily medication, a peak flow meter may not be useful for asthma management.

Why should I measure my peak flow rate?

Measurements with a peak flow meter can help you and your health care provider monitor your asthma. These measurements can be important

About This Chapter: Text in this chapter is from "Peak Flow Meters," © 2009 American Lung Association. Reprinted with permission. For more information about the American Lung Association or to support the work it does, call 800-LUNG-USA (800-586-4872) or log on to www.LungUSA.org.

and help your health care provider pre-scribe medicines to keep your asthma in control.

A peak flow meter can show you that you may need to change the way you are using your medicines. For example, peak flow readings may help be a signal for you to implement the medication plan you and your health care provider have developed for worsening asthma.

On the other hand, if you are doing well, then measuring your peak flow may be helpful as you and your health care provider try to lower the level of your medicines.

☞ Remember!!

A peak flow meter can also be used during an asthma epi-sode. It can help you determine the severity of the episode; decide when to use your rescue medication; and decide when to seek emergency care.

Knowing your "personal" peak flow rate allows you to evaluate your readings. Be-ing at your "best" can provide reassur-ance and make you feel more self-confident.

Source: Reprinted with permission. © 2009 American Lung Association.

A peak flow meter can help you when your asthma is getting worse. Asthma sometimes changes gradually. Your peak flow may show changes before you feel them. It can allow your health care provider to adjust your treatment to prevent urgent calls to the health care provider, emergency room visits, or hospitalizations.

How do you use a peak flow meter?

Step 1: Before each use, make sure the sliding marker or arrow on the Peak Flow Meter is at the bottom of the numbered scale (zero or the lowest number on the scale).

Step 2: Stand up straight. Remove gum or any food from your mouth. Take a deep breath (as deep as you can). Put the mouthpiece of the peak flow meter into your mouth. Close your lips tightly around the mouthpiece. Be sure to keep your tongue away from the mouthpiece. In one breath blow out as hard and as quickly as possible. Blow a "fast hard blast" rather than "slowly blowing" until you have emptied out nearly all of the air from your lungs.

Step 3: The force of the air coming out of your lungs causes the marker to move along the numbered scale. Note the number on a piece of paper.

Step 4: Repeat the entire routine three times. (You know you have done the routine correctly when the numbers from all three tries are very close together.)

Step 5: Record the highest of the three ratings. Do not calculate an average. This is very important. You can't breathe out too much when using your peak flow meter but you can breathe out too little. Record your highest reading.

Step 6: Measure your peak flow rate close to the same time each day. You and your health care provider can determine the best times. One suggestion is to measure your peak flow rate twice daily between 7 and 9 a.m. and between 6 and 8 p.m.

You may want to measure your peak flow rate before or after using your medicine. Some people measure peak flow both before and after taking medication. Try to do it the same way each time.

Step 7: Keep a chart of your peak flow rates. Discuss the readings with your health care provider.

Name _____ Week Beginning (Date) _____
Peak Flow Zones: Green Zone _____ Yellow Zone _____ Red Zone: _____
Prescribed Medications (include dose and frequency) _____

Peak Flow Recording Times. _____ AM _____ PM

Day	Sunday		Monday		Tuesday		Wednesday		Thursday		Friday		Saturday	
Time	AM	PM	AM	PM	AM	PM	AM	PM	AM	PM	AM	PM	AM	PM
600														
550														
500														
450														
400														
350														
300														
250														
200														
150														
100														
Changes in Medicine														
Notes														

(Your Peak Flow Rates (liters/minute))

Figure 16.1. Peak Flow Chart—Sample Chart

How can I determine a "normal" peak flow rate for me?

Three zones of measurement are commonly used to interpret peak flow rates. It is easy to relate the three zones to the traffic light colors: green, yellow, and red. In general, a normal peak flow rate can vary as much as 20 percent.

Be aware of the following general guidelines. Keep in mind that recognizing changes from "normal" is important. Your health care provider may suggest other zones to follow.

> **✔ Quick Tip**
>
> Discuss the use of a peak flow meter with your health care provider. Make measuring your peak flow rate a part of your personal asthma management program.
>
> Source: Reprinted with permission. © 2009 American Lung Association.

Green Zone: 80 to 100 percent of your usual or "normal" peak flow rate signals all clear. A reading in this zone means that your asthma is under reasonably good control. It would be advisable to continue your prescribed program of management.

Yellow Zone: 50 to 80 percent of your usual or "normal" peak flow rate signals caution. It is a time for decisions. Your airways are narrowing and may require extra treatment. Your symptoms can get better or worse depending on what you do, or how and when you use your prescribed medication. You and your health care provider should have a plan for yellow zone readings.

Red Zone: Less than 50 percent of your usual or "normal" peak flow rate signals a Medical Alert. Immediate decisions and actions need to be taken. Severe airway narrowing may be occurring. Take your rescue medications right away. Contact your health care provider now and follow the plan he has given you for red zone readings.

Some health care providers may suggest zones with a smaller range such as 90 to 100 percent. Always follow your health care provider's suggestions about your peak flow rate.

Source: Reprinted with permission. © 2009 American Lung Association.

Chapter 17

Tips For Controlling Your Asthma

Take Control Of Asthma

New Guidelines from the National Heart, Lung and Blood Institute (NHLBI)'s National Asthma Education and Prevention Program use the latest research to help you take control of your asthma symptoms and reduce the effects of the disease on your life. Your goal should be to feel good, be active all day and sleep well at night. All patients with asthma should accept nothing less.

If your asthma is in control, you should expect:

- no or few asthma symptoms, even at night or after exercise;
- prevention of all or most asthma attacks;
- participation in all activities, including exercise;
- no emergency room visits or hospital stays;
- less need for quick-relief medicines;
- no or few side effects from medicines.

Keep Asthma Symptoms In Check

Many of the 22 million Americans who have asthma limit their activities and miss work or school. The disease also can kill. Almost 4,000 people die from asthma each year and most of these deaths are preventable. Uncontrolled asthma and asthma deaths happen when the disease is not treated correctly or sometimes because people do not know they have asthma.

Effective asthma treatment begins with the right diagnosis early in the disease. Delays can lead to permanent lung damage.

Your doctor first decides how to treat your asthma by looking at what your symptoms are now and what they have been in the past. The doctor also will try to determine your risk for future attacks. This information will help you and your doctor develop a plan to manage your disease and keep your asthma under control.

If you just started treatment or have frequent symptoms, your doctor may want to see you every two to six weeks. Once treatment is under way, doctor visits may be every one to six months to check asthma control, even when you have no symptoms.

During your visits, the doctor will review your symptoms, activities and medicines. Between visits, it is important for you to monitor your asthma by keeping an asthma diary to track your symptoms or using a peak flow meter to measure the air flow from your lungs. With either method, you also should keep track of your medication use. This information will help you and your doctor decide if any changes in your treatment plan are needed.

Avoid Asthma Triggers

Often the best way to control asthma symptoms is to stay away from whatever causes or "triggers" them. Asthma triggers frequently include:

- things to which you are allergic (allergens) such as pollen, dust mites, cockroaches, molds, and animal danders;

- tobacco smoke, air pollution, formaldehyde, and other volatile organic substances;

- medicines such as aspirin and acetaminophen;
- cold air;
- exercise.

Some health problems also can trigger or make asthma symptoms worse. These include obesity, obstructive sleep apnea, acid reflux, the common cold, sinus infections, stress, and depression. Let your doctor know if you have one of these conditions so you can discuss the best approach to control both your health problem and your asthma symptoms.

Use Proper Asthma Medication

Today, there are many effective medicines to treat asthma. Most people with asthma need two kinds.

✔ Quick Tip
Partner With Your Doctor

Your doctor is your partner in learning about and managing your asthma. Together, you and your doctor should:

- talk about your treatment goals and how you can reach them;
- develop a written asthma action plan that explains the treatment you need every day and what to do if your symptoms become worse;
- review your asthma medicines so that you understand the purpose of each;
- practice how to take your medicine;
- discuss how to keep track of your symptoms and make decisions about how much medicine to take;
- review the things that make your asthma worse—your "asthma triggers"—and discuss tips on how to avoid them.

The more you learn about your asthma and your medicines that treat it, the more you can keep your disease in control.

Quick-Relief Medicines: These medicines are taken at the first sign of any asthma symptoms for immediate relief:

- Short-acting inhaled beta2-agonists

- Anticholinergics

Your doctor also may recommend you use these medicines before exercise. Quick-relief medicines can stop asthma symptoms, but they do not control airway inflammation that causes the symptoms. If you find that you need your quick-relief medicine to treat asthma symptoms more than twice a week, or two or more nights a month, then your asthma is not well controlled. Be sure to tell you doctor.

Long-Term Control Medicines: These medicines are taken every day to prevent symptoms and attacks:

- Antileukotrienes or leukotriene modifiers

- Cromolyn sodium and nedocromil

- Inhaled corticosteroids

- Long-acting inhaled beta2-agonists (never taken alone)

- Methylxanthines

- Oral corticosteroids

- Immunomodulators

> ✔ **Quick Tip**
> **Consider**
> **Allergy Shots**
>
> If you cannot avoid an allergic asthma trigger and you have symptoms three days a week and more than two nights a month, you should consider allergy shots. Also known as immunotherapy, the shots are especially helpful when symptoms occur year-round or are not easily controlled by medicine.

These medicines are taken every day even if you do not have symptoms. The most effective long-term control medicines reduce airway inflammation and help improve asthma control.

Your doctor will work with you to find the right medicine, or combination of medicines, to manage your asthma, and will adjust the type and amount based on your symptoms and control. The goal is to have you feel your best with the least amount of medicine.

See An Allergist, An Asthma Specialist

An allergist can help you learn more about your asthma and develop a treatment plan that works for you.

The Guidelines say that you should see an asthma specialist if you:

- have asthma symptoms every day and often at night that cause you to limit your activity;

- have had a life-threatening asthma attack;

- do not meet the goals of your asthma treatment after three to six months, or your doctor believes you are not responding to current treatment;

- have symptoms that are unusual or hard to diagnose;

- have conditions such as severe hay fever or sinusitis that complicate your asthma or your diagnosis;

- need more tests to find out more about your asthma and the causes of your symptoms;

- need more help and instruction on your treatment plan, medicines, or asthma triggers;

- might be helped by allergy shots;

- need oral corticosteroid therapy or high-dose inhaled corticosteroids;

- have taken oral corticosteroids more than twice in one year;

- have stayed in a hospital because of your asthma;

- need help to identify your asthma triggers.

☞ Remember!!

An asthma specialist is recommended for children ages 0–4 who have asthma symptoms every day and three to four nights or more a month, and should be considered for children who have symptoms three days or more a week and one to two nights a month.

Chapter 18

Asthma Attacks

What's An Asthma Flare-Up?

For someone with asthma, the airways in the lungs are a problem. They're always a little swollen or irritated, but during an asthma flare-up (also called an asthma flare, attack, episode, or exacerbation), the problems worsen. Sticky mucus clogs these important tubes. And the muscles around the airways tighten up, further narrowing the airway. This leaves very little room inside for the air to flow through. Think of a straw with walls that are getting thicker and narrower, leaving less and less space inside for air to get through.

A flare-up can cause coughing, chest tightness, wheezing, and trouble breathing. A person having a flare-up also might sweat or feel his or her heart beating faster. If the flare-up is severe, the person may struggle to breathe even while sitting still. He or she may not be able to speak more than few words at a time without pausing for breath.

Because they can be life threatening, all asthma flare-ups demand attention. Someone having an asthma flare-up might need to take rescue medication, visit

About This Chapter: Text in this chapter is from "What's an Asthma Flare-Up?" March 2007, reprinted with permission from www.kidshealth.org. Copyright © 2007 The Nemours Foundation. This information was provided by KidsHealth, one of the largest resources online for medically reviewed health information written for parents, kids, and teens. For more articles like this one, visit www.KidsHealth.org, or www.TeensHealth.org.

the doctor, or even go to the hospital. Having a set of instructions called an asthma action plan can help you know which course of action is needed.

Flare-Up Causes

Certain things can bring on symptoms in someone who has asthma. These are known as triggers. It may not always be clear what a person's triggers are, but common triggers include tobacco smoke, cold air, exercise, and infections, such as colds.

A lot of people who have asthma also have allergies. In these people, the allergens—the things that cause the allergic symptoms—can also cause asthma flare-ups. Examples of common allergic triggers include animal dander, dust mites, mold, and cockroaches.

Exposure to a trigger can lead to an asthma flare-up in several ways. It can worsen the swelling in the airways and increase the amount of mucus made there. It can also cause the muscles around the airways to tighten, making the airways even narrower.

Left untreated, a flare-up can last for several hours or even several days. Rescue medications often take care of the symptoms pretty quickly, and most people feel better once the flare-up is over, although it can take several days to completely clear up.

✎ What's It Mean?

Airway: Any part of the respiratory tract through which air passes during breathing.

Allergen: Term for an antigen that induces an allergic or hypersensitive response.

Asthma: An inflammatory disease of the lungs characterized by reversible (in most cases) airway obstruction. Originally, a term used to mean "difficult breathing"; now used to denote bronchial asthma. (Synonym: reactive airway disease.)

Bronchi: Two subdivisions of the trachea serving to convey air to and from the lungs. The trachea divides into right and left main bronchi, which in turn form lobar, segmental, and intrasegmental bronchi. (The singular form is bronchus.)

Bronchia: The smaller divisions of the bronchi (Synonym: bronchial tubes).

Trigger: Term describing a system in which a relatively small input turns on a relatively large output, the magnitude of which is unrelated to the magnitude of the input.

Source: From *Stedman's Medical Dictionary, 27th Edition*, copyright © 2000 Lippincott Williams & Wilkins. All rights reserved.

Can You Predict A Flare-Up?

Flare-ups vary a lot from person to person and even from attack to attack. Some flare-ups happen suddenly, when a person has been exposed to a trigger, such as tobacco smoke. But other flare-ups happen because problems in the airways have been building up over time, especially in people whose asthma is not well controlled.

✎ What's It Mean?

Asthma Action Plan: The asthma action plan shows your daily treatment, such as what kind of medicines to take and when to take them. The plan explains when to call the doctor or go to the emergency room.

Asthma Flare-Up: Asthma attacks also are called flare-ups or exacerbations. When the airways react, the muscles around them tighten. This causes the airways to narrow, and less air flows to your lungs. The swelling also can worsen, making the airways even narrower. Cells in the airways may make more mucus than normal. Mucus is a sticky, thick liquid that can further narrow your airways. This chain reaction can result in asthma symptoms. Sometimes symptoms are mild and go away on their own or after minimal treatment with an asthma medicine. At other times, symptoms continue to get worse. When symptoms get more intense and/or additional symptoms appear, this is an asthma attack.

Control Medications: Long-term control medicines help reduce airway inflammation and prevent asthma symptoms.

Peak Flow Meter: This is small, hand-held device that shows how well air moves out of your lungs. You blow into the device and it gives you a score, or peak flow number. Your score shows how well your lungs are working at the time of the test.

Rescue Medications: Quick-relief, or "rescue," medicines relieve asthma symptoms that may flare up.

Source: Excerpted from "Asthma," *Diseases and Conditions Index*, National Heart Lung and Blood Institute (www.nhlbi.nih.gov), September 2008.

Flare-ups can and should be treated at their earliest stages, so it's important to recognize early warning signs. These are things that a person might experience just before a flare-up occurs. These clues are unique to each person and may be the same or different with each asthma flare-up. Early warning signs include:

- coughing, even if you don't have a cold;

- throat clearing;

- rapid or irregular breathing;

- unusual fatigue;

- restless sleep;

- difficulty with exercise.

A peak flow meter also can be a useful tool in predicting whether a flare-up is on its way.

Preventing Flare-Ups

You also have the power to prevent flare-ups, at least some of the time. Here's what you can do:

- Always have your inhaler and spacer with you.

- Stay away from triggers that you know may cause flare-ups.

- Take your controller medicine as directed. Don't skip it or take less of it because you are feeling better.

- Work with your parents and doctor to follow an asthma action plan.

Part Three

Medications Used To Treat Asthma Symptoms

Chapter 19

How Is Asthma Treated?

What's The Difference Between Rescue And Controller Medications?

Asthma medicine comes in two main types: controller medicine and rescue medicine. Rescue medications, also called quick-relief or fast-acting medications, work immediately to relieve asthma symptoms when they occur. These types of medicines are often inhaled directly into the lungs, where they open up the airways and relieve symptoms such as wheezing, coughing, and shortness of breath, often within minutes. But as effective as they are, rescue medications don't have a long-term effect.

Controller medications, also called *preventive* or *maintenance* medications, work over a period of time to reduce airway inflammation and help prevent asthma symptoms from occurring. They may be inhaled or swallowed as a pill or liquid.

Rescue Medications

Quick-acting bronchodilators, usually given through an inhaler or a nebulizer, loosen the tightened muscles around inflamed airways and are the most often-prescribed rescue medications. The most common of these are called beta2-agonists. These medications are related to adrenaline and usually work within minutes to provide temporary relief of symptoms.

If the bronchodilator alone doesn't resolve a severe flare-up, other medications may be given by mouth or injection to help treat it.

If you have been prescribed rescue medication, it's important to keep these medicines on hand. That means at home, at the mall, at sport practice, and even on vacation.

> ✎ **What's It Mean?**
>
> <u>Controller Medicine</u>: Controller medications, also called *preventive* or *maintenance* medications, work over a period of time to reduce airway inflammation and help prevent asthma symptoms from occurring.
>
> <u>Rescue Medicine</u>: Rescue medications, also called *quick-relief* or *fast-acting* medications, work immediately to relieve asthma symptoms when they occur.
>
> Source: © May 2007 The Nemours Foundation.

Rescue medications, although an important part of asthma treatment, can be overused. Talk with your doctor about how often you use the rescue medication. If it's too much, the doctor also may prescribe a controller medicine, designed to prevent asthma flare-ups from happening.

Controller Medications

Because your airways may be inflamed even in between flare-ups, controller medications may be needed to prevent unexpected asthma flare-ups. Slower-acting controller medicines can take days to weeks to start working, but when they do, they prevent airway inflammation and keep the lungs from making too much mucus.

There are a variety of controller medications, but inhaled corticosteroids are most common. They're usually given through an inhaler or nebulizer. Despite their name, corticosteroids are not the same as performance-enhancing steroids used by athletes. They are a safe and proven form of treatment for asthma.

In fact, inhaled corticosteroids are the preferred long-term treatment for children with frequent asthma symptoms. Research shows that they improve asthma control and their risk of causing long-term negative effects is minimal. (But corticosteroids that are swallowed in liquid or pill form may cause side effects if used daily over a long period of time.)

Long-acting bronchodilators can also be used as controller medications. These relax the muscles of the airways for up to 12 hours, but can't be used for quick relief of symptoms because they don't start to work immediately.

Even if you take controller medicine regularly, rescue medication will still be needed to handle flare-ups when they occur.

Working With The Doctor

Your doctor will determine which type of medicine you need, depending on how frequent and how severe the asthma symptoms are. Both the type and dosage of medication that you need are likely to change, with the goal being to have you on the lowest amount of medication necessary for effective asthma management.

You're an important player in your asthma treatment. For example, you can track how well the medicine is working by using a peak flow meter. You also can record information in an asthma diary and ask your doctor to create an asthma action plan, if you don't already have one. By reporting any concerns or changes in your symptoms, you can provide information that will help the doctor select the best course of treatment.

What's An Asthma Action Plan?

Source: From "What's an Asthma Action Plan?" June 2007, reprinted with permission from www.kidshealth.org. Copyright © 2007 The Nemours Foundation. This information was provided by KidsHealth, one of the largest resources online for medically reviewed health information written for parents, kids, and teens. For more articles like www.KidsHealth.org, or www.TeensHealth.org.

What Is It?

An asthma action plan, or management plan, is a written plan that you develop with your doctor. It is designed to help you take control of your asthma, so it doesn't get in the way of playing sports, working out, going to parties, or doing whatever you want to do.

Following an asthma action plan will help you prevent flare-ups and deal with the ones you can't prevent. Knowing how to deal with flare-ups can keep you from having to visit the emergency department.

Your doctor may give you an action plan, or you can print out a sample one and ask him or her to help you complete it. Having a written, step-by-step plan means that you don't have to memorize everything your doctor said. You can keep a copy with you at all times or choose to memorize key parts of it.

Your asthma action plan will give you clear instructions so you can:

- avoid triggers that worsen your asthma;
- notice early symptoms of a flare-up and treat them;
- take the right steps to deal with an asthma flare-up;
- know when to seek emergency care.

Action Plans Are Individual

Asthma varies from person to person, so there isn't a one-size-fits-all asthma action plan. Each plan will be somewhat different, but a key part of any action plan will detail what you need to do during a flare-up. It will tell you when you need to take your rescue medication, how much to take in different circumstances, and when it's time to call the doctor or go to the emergency department for care.

Many action plans use the "zone system," which is based on the colors of a traffic light. This is the same color system used on peak flow meters. Action plans use symptoms, peak flow readings, or both to help you determine what zone your asthma is in:

- The green zone, or safety zone, explains how to manage your asthma on a daily basis, when you're feeling good.

- The yellow zone, or caution zone, explains how to look for signs that your asthma is getting worse. It also instructs you on which medications to add to bring your asthma back under control.

- The red zone, or danger zone, explains what to do when a flare-up is severe.

The color system makes it easy to figure out which instructions apply to you based on your peak flow meter reading. Your "personal best" peak flow reading is an important measurement to include on the plan, so you'll have something to compare the new numbers to.

In addition to information about flare-ups, your action plan may include:

- emergency phone numbers and locations of emergency care facilities;

☞ Remember!!
Understand Your Plan

For your asthma action plan to be effective, you have to follow it, even when you are feeling OK. That means you need to understand it and it needs to fit realistically into your life. For example, if exercise is one of your triggers, you need to talk with your doctor about your sport and workouts.

Review your plan with your doctor and make sure you understand it. Ask questions. Talk with your doctor about ideas you have for making the plan work better for you. For example, your doctor might be willing to adjust the time of day that you take your asthma medicine to better fit into your schedule.

And if you've been following an asthma action plan but it doesn't seem to be controlling your asthma as well as it used to, let your doctor know. He or she may need to make some adjustments in your medication or other aspects of your plan. Also tell your doctor if you don't seem to need your rescue medication as much any more. If your asthma is well controlled, your doctor might reduce the amount of controller medicine you're taking.

Source: © June 2007
The Nemours Foundation.

- a list of triggers and how to avoid them;

- steps to take before exercising;

- a list of early flare-up symptoms to watch for and what to do when they occur;

- the names and dosages of all your medications and when and how they should be used.

Chapter 20

Understanding The Different Types Of Asthma Medications

Can medicine cure my asthma?

No, there is no cure for asthma. Although asthma cannot be cured it can be controlled. There are many medicines that help people with asthma. Some are preventive medicines and others are known as quick relievers. The preventive medicines are used for long-term control of the disease and work to make asthma attacks less frequent and less severe. Quick reliever medicines offer short-term relief of symptoms when asthma episodes occur.

Unless your asthma is very mild, chances are you have prescriptions for at least two different medicines. That can be confusing. The more you understand about what those medicines do and why they help, the more likely you are to use them correctly.

Although there are some potential unfavorable side effects from taking asthma medications, the benefit of successfully controlling your asthma outweighs the risks. It is important to discuss each of your asthma medications with your physician to learn more about their effects.

As just discussed, there are two kinds of asthma medications: long-term controllers and quick relievers.

Long-Term Control Medicines: Standard asthma treatment begins with long-term relief from anti-inflammatory drugs. These drugs make the airways less sensitive, and keeps them from reacting as easily to triggers. They reduce coughing, wheezing and the struggle for breath, and they allow you to live an active life. To have long-term control of your asthma depends on you. Anti-inflammatory drugs must be taken exactly as they are prescribed.

- *Cromolyn Sodium* (Inhaled: Intal) and *Nedocromil Sodium* (Inhaled: Tilade) prevent airways from swelling when they come in contact with asthma triggers. These non-steroids can also be used to prevent asthma caused by exercise.

- *Inhaled Corticosteroids* (AeroBid, Azmacort, Beclovent, Flovent, Pulmicort, Vanceril) prevent and reduce airway swelling and decrease the amount of mucus in the lungs. These are generally safe when taken as directed. They are not the same as anabolic steroids, which some athletes take to build muscles. If you are taking an inhaled anti-inflammatory medicine and you feel your asthma symptoms getting worse, talk with your doctor about continuing or increasing the medicine that you are already taking. You may also need to add an oral corticosteroid or a short-acting beta antagonist (bronchodilator) for relief.

- *Oral Corticosteroids* (Pills or tablets: Aristocort, Celestone, Decadron, Medrol, Prednisone, Sterapred) (Liquid for children: Pediapred, Prelone) are used as short-term treatment for severe asthma episodes or as long-term therapy for some people with severe asthma. Again, these are not the same as anabolic steroids.

- *Long-acting beta agonists* (Inhaled: Serevent) can be taken with or without an anti-inflammatory medicine to help control daily symptoms, including nighttime asthma. This type of medicine can also prevent asthma triggered by exercise. Because long-acting beta agonists can not relieve symptoms quickly, they should not be used for an acute attack. You also need a short-acting, inhaled beta agonist for acute symptoms. Long-acting, inhaled beta agonists are not a substitute for anti-inflammatory medicine. You should not decrease or stop taking your anti-inflammatory medicine without talking to your doctor, even if you feel better.

- *Leukotriene modifiers* (Tablets: Accolate, Singulair) are a new type of long-term control medication. They prevent airway inflammation and swelling, decrease the amount of mucus in the lungs, and open the airways.

- *Combined therapy medicine* (inhaled) contains both a controller and reliever medicine. This combination of a long-acting bronchodilator and corticosteroid is used for long-term control.

- *Anti-IgE therapy* (injected) is a new treatment for people with moderate or severe allergic asthma. It attempts to stop allergic asthma at its root cause instead of just treating asthma symptoms. This drug is not inhaled, but rather injected by your doctor on a regular basis. It does not eliminate your need for other asthma medications, but it can help to reduce your use of them. Due to its significant cost, this form of therapy is currently reserved for moderate to severe cases requiring multiple medications.

Quick Relief Medicines: These medicines ease the wheezing, coughing and tightness of the chest that occurs during asthma episodes.

- *Short-acting bronchodilators* are one type of quick relief medicine. They open airways by relaxing muscles that tighten in and around the airways during asthma episodes.

- *Short-acting beta agonists* (Inhaled: Albuterol, Alupent, Brethaire, Bronkosol, Isoetharine, Maxair, Medihaler-Iso, Metaprel, Proventil, Tornalate, Ventolin, Xopenex) relieve asthma symptoms quickly and some prevent asthma caused by exercise. If you use one of these medicines every day, or if you use it more than three times in a single day, your asthma may be getting worse, or you may not be using your inhaler correctly. Talk with your doctor right away about adding or increasing a medication, and about your inhaler technique.

- *Oral beta agonists* (Syrup, tablets, and long-acting tablets: Alupent, Brethine, Bricanyl, Proventil, Proventil Repetabs, Ventolin, Volmax).

Syrup may be used for children, while long-acting tablets may be used for nighttime asthma. Oral preparations generally cause more side effects than the inhaled form.

- *Theophylline* (Oral, slow acting: Aerolate, Elixophyllin, Quibron-T, Resbid, Slo-bid, T-Phyl, Theolair, Theo-24, Theo-Dur, Theo-X, Uni-Dur, Uniphyl) can be used for persistently symptomatic asthma, and especially to prevent nighttime asthma. Theophylline must remain at a constant level in the blood stream to be effective. Too high a level can be dangerous. Your doctor will do regular blood tests. Sustained release Theophylline is not the preferred primary long-term control treatment, but it is effective when added to other anti-inflammatory medicines to control nighttime episodes.

Can medicine alone help my asthma?

No. Although medicines help a lot, you cannot expect them to do the job alone. *You* have to help. You have to avoid the things that cause (or trigger) your asthma symptoms as much as you can, even if they are things you like. In planning to avoid these triggers, you need to think about outdoor exposure as well as the things at home and at work that cause your problem.

Will I always have to take the same amount of medicine?

Not necessarily. You will probably take most when you begin treatment, while your doctor learns what causes your asthma, which medicine(s) control it most effectively and at what doses. Once this is completed, your medications may be reduced in number, frequency or dose. The goal of this "step-down" method is

☞ **Remember!!**

The job of these medicines is to control your asthma in both normal and stressful situations so that your airways remain open and your lungs operate properly. This enables you to live an active life free from fear of struggling for breath. But for the medicines to do their best work, you must understand your condition, know what your medicines can and cannot do, and use them exactly as instructed by your doctor.

Your intelligent use of asthma medicines is as important as the medicines themselves.

to gain control of your asthma as quickly as possible, then maintain effective control with as little medication as necessary. Once long-term, anti-inflammatory therapy has begun, proper monitoring requires examination by a doctor every 1 to 6 months.

Will I have to take medicine all the time?

Not necessarily. Because asthma is a chronic condition that is controllable but currently can not be cured, you will have asthma all the time even if you are symptom free much of the time. Your medical treatment will take into consideration the severity and frequency of your symptoms. If you have little inflammation between episodes, and if the episodes are infrequent, your treatment will emphasize quick relief from acute symptoms, particularly if they are mild.

If your symptoms occur at certain times and from a known and predictable cause, you will be treated accordingly. If, for example, you have "seasonal asthma" because of an allergy to a specific pollen, you may take medicines only when that pollen is in the air. But asthma so specific is uncommon, and most people with asthma take some form of medication most or all of the time.

Will medicine help me sleep better?

Yes. It is common for asthma symptoms to occur at night, and many people tell of the panic of awakening in a struggle for breath. These nighttime symptoms can be controlled with asthma medicines taken on a regular basis.

In addition, some bedding materials may be among your allergens, and must be replaced with non-allergenic materials. Air filters in your bedroom may also help to maximize the benefits of your medicines if you have nighttime symptoms of asthma.

Will medicines help me breathe better when I exercise?

Yes. Physical activity, especially when combined with an irritant like cold air, may cause your airways to open and close irregularly. This is called exertion-induced bronchospasm (EBI). The short-term-relief asthma medicines, taken before and during exercise, usually control this. Thanks to these medicines, many Olympic and professional athletes enjoy successful sports careers despite their asthma.

☞ Remember!!
Do asthma drugs have side effects?

Yes, as do all drugs. No medicine is so exact that it can do its intended job without having unintended side effects as well. It is important, therefore, that you give your doctor accurate information about your entire health condition, not just your asthma symptoms. Doing away with some asthma drugs on the basis of other health problems, like high blood pressure, is one important way of reducing your risks.

For most people with asthma, long-term control of inflammation of the airways is the key to successful treatment. Prescribing drugs based on information you supply is your doctor's responsibility. Faithful reporting of changes and reactions is yours. And only you can make sure that you take your medication exactly as it is prescribed.

The greatest danger for most people taking asthma medicine, especially by inhaler, is *overuse*. Don't give in to "just another puff," or "if two puffs work, three must be better," or "half a dose between doses." Overuse of these medications over a period of years may prove to be very harmful.

Your doctor, your pharmacist, and the medicine's label will tell you exactly the frequency and amount of your doses. Do not exceed them without your doctor's instructions. If either your doctor or pharmacist says that "you are going through this awfully quickly," you are almost certainly overusing. Overusing is overdosing.

Chapter 21

What You Need To Know About Anti-IgE Treatment

Why is this medication prescribed?

Omalizumab injection is used to decrease the number of asthma attacks (sudden episodes of wheezing, shortness of breath, and trouble breathing) in people with allergic asthma (asthma caused by inhaling substances such as dander, pollen, and dust mites) whose symptoms are not controlled with inhaled steroids. Omalizumab is in a class of medications called monoclonal antibodies. It works by blocking the action of immunoglobulin E (IgE), a natural substance in the body that causes the symptoms of allergic asthma.

How should this medicine be used?

Omalizumab injection comes as a solution (liquid) to inject subcutaneously (under the skin). It is usually injected in a doctor's office once every two weeks or every four weeks. You may receive one or more injections at each visit, depending on the dose prescribed by your doctor.

It may take some time before you feel the full benefit of omalizumab. Call your doctor if your asthma symptoms worsen. Talk to your doctor so that you know what to do if you have an asthma attack or breathing problems while using omalizumab. Omalizumab will not relieve the symptoms of a sudden asthma attack.

Omalizumab injection may be used along with other medications for asthma. Do not decrease your dose of any other asthma medication or stop taking any other asthma medication that has been prescribed by your doctor, unless your doctor tells you to do so. Your doctor may want to decrease your dose of some other asthma medications gradually.

> ♣ **It's A Fact!!**
> **Other Uses For**
> **This Medicine**
>
> This medication may be prescribed for other uses; ask your doctor or pharmacist for more information.
>
> Source: © 2009 American Society of Health-System Pharmacists, Inc.

What special precautions should I follow?

Before using omalizumab injection,

- tell your doctor and pharmacist if you are allergic to any medications;

- tell your doctor and pharmacist what prescription and nonprescription medications, vitamins, nutritional supplements, and herbal products you are taking or plan to take;

- tell your doctor if you have any other medical conditions and if you are being treated with allergy immunotherapy (allergy shots; a series of injections given regularly to prevent the body from developing allergic reactions to specific substances);

- tell your doctor if you are pregnant, plan to become pregnant, or are breast-feeding. If you become pregnant while using omalizumab, call your doctor.

- talk to your doctor about whether there is a risk that you will develop a hookworm, roundworm, whipworm, or threadworm infection (infection with worms that live inside the body). If you are at high risk of developing this type of infection, using omalizumab may increase the chance that you will actually become infected. Most of these infections are rare in the United States, but if you are at risk of developing an infection, your doctor can suggest ways to prevent infection and will monitor you carefully during your treatment.

What special dietary instructions should I follow?

Unless your doctor tells you otherwise, continue your normal diet.

🖐 Remember!!
Important Warning

Omalizumab injection may cause a serious or life-threatening allergic reaction. An allergic reaction may occur immediately after an injection of omalizumab is given or 24 hours or longer after the injection is given. People who did not have an allergic reaction to their first dose of omalizumab may have an allergic reaction after they receive another dose of the medication.

Tell your doctor if you have ever had an allergic reaction after receiving an injection of omalizumab. You should not receive omalizumab injection if you have ever had an allergic reaction to the medication.

You will receive each injection of omalizumab in your doctor's office. You will stay in the office for some time after you receive the medication so your doctor can watch you closely. Tell your doctor if you experience any of the following symptoms of an allergic reaction: wheezing or difficulty breathing, shortness of breath, cough, chest tightness, dizziness, fainting, fast or weak heartbeat, anxiety, feeling that something bad is about to happen, flushing, itching, hives, feeling warm, swelling of the throat or tongue, throat tightness, hoarse voice, or difficulty swallowing. Get immediate emergency medical attention if you experience any of these symptoms after you leave your doctor's office.

Your doctor will give you the manufacturer's patient information sheet (Medication Guide) each time you receive an injection of omalizumab. Read the information carefully and ask your doctor or pharmacist if you have any questions. You can also visit the Food and Drug Administration (FDA) website (http://www.fda.gov/cder) or the manufacturer's website to obtain the Medication Guide.

Talk to your doctor about the risks of using omalizumab.

Source: © 2009 American Society of Health-System Pharmacists, Inc.

What should I do if I forget a dose?

If you miss an appointment to receive an injection of omalizumab, you should call your doctor as soon as possible. The missed dose should be given as soon as it can be rescheduled.

What side effects can this medication cause?

Omalizumab injection may cause side effects. Tell your doctor if any of these symptoms are severe or do not go away:

- Pain, redness, swelling, warmth, burning, stinging, bruising, hardness (bump), or itching in the place omalizumab was injected

- Pain, especially in the joints, arms, or legs

- Tiredness

- Ear pain

Omalizumab may increase the risk of developing cancer, including breast, skin, parotid (salivary gland, located near the mouth), and prostate cancer. Talk to your doctor about the risks of using this medication.

Omalizumab may cause other side effects. Call your doctor if you have any unusual problems while using this medication.

If you experience a serious side effect, you or your doctor may send a report to the Food and Drug Administration's (FDA) MedWatch Adverse Event Reporting program online at http://www.fda.gov/MedWatch/index.html or by phone: 1-800-332-1088.

What storage conditions are needed for this medicine?

Your doctor will store this medication in his or her office.

What other information should I know?

Keep all appointments with your doctor.

Before having any laboratory test, tell your doctor and the laboratory personnel that you are taking or have taken omalizumab.

☞ Remember!!
Xolair (omalizumab) Safety Alerts

July 2, 2007: Genetech and FDA informed healthcare professionals and asthmatic patients that the prescribing information for Xolair was revised to include a new BOXED WARNING, and updated WARNINGS, PRECAUTIONS, and ADVERSE REACTIONS sections that address the risk of anaphylaxis (the onset of action can be delayed for 24 hours or more) when taking this medication. In addition, a new MEDICATION GUIDE was developed and will be provided to patients when a prescription for Xolair is filled or re-filled at the pharmacy. Due to the risk of anaphylaxis, Xolair should only be administered to patients in a healthcare setting under direct medical supervision. Patients should be observed for an appropriate period of time following each Xolair injection.

February 21, 2007: FDA notified asthmatic patients and healthcare professionals of new reports of serious and life-threatening allergic reactions (anaphylaxis) in patients after treatment with Xolair (omalizumab). Usually these reactions occur within two hours of receiving a Xolair subcutaneous injection. However, these new reports include patients who had delayed anaphylaxis—with onset two to 24 hours or even longer—after receiving Xolair treatment. Anaphylaxis may occur after any dose of Xolair (including the first dose), even if the patient had no allergic reaction to the first dose. Health care professionals who administer Xolair should be prepared to manage life-threatening anaphylaxis and should observe their Xolair-treated patients for at least two hours after Xolair is given. Patients under treatment with Xolair should be fully informed about the signs and symptoms of anaphylaxis, their chance of developing delayed anaphylaxis following Xolair treatment, and how to treat it when it occurs. FDA has requested Genetech add a boxed warning to the product label and to revise the Xolair label and provide a MEDICATION GUIDE for patients to strengthen the existing warning for anaphylaxis.

Source: "Safety: Xolair (Omalizumab),"
U.S. Food and Drug Administration, 2007.

It is important for you to keep a written list of all of the prescription and nonprescription (over-the-counter) medicines you are taking, as well as any products such as vitamins, minerals, or other dietary supplements. You should bring this list with you each time you visit a doctor or if you are admitted to a hospital. It is also important information to carry with you in case of emergencies.

Brand Names: Xolair®

✔ **Quick Tip**
In Case Of
Emergency/Overdose

In case of overdose, call your local poison control center at 1-800-222-1222. If the victim has collapsed or is not breathing, call local emergency services at 911.

Source: © 2009 American Society of Health-System Pharmacists, Inc.

Chapter 22

What You Need To Know About Bronchodilators

Treating Asthma With Bronchodilators

Bronchodilators relieve asthma symptoms by relaxing the muscle bands that tighten around the airways. This action rapidly opens the airways, letting more air come in and out of the lungs. As a result, breathing improves. Bronchodilators also help clear mucus from the lungs. As the airways open, the mucus moves more freely and can be coughed out more easily.

In short-acting forms, bronchodilators *relieve* or *stop* asthma symptoms and are very helpful during an asthma attack. In long-acting forms, bronchodilators help control asthma symptoms and prevent asthma attacks.

There are two main types of bronchodilator medicines: beta 2-agonists (short- and long-acting forms) and anticholinergics.

Beta 2-agonists—short-acting inhaled forms include:

About This Chapter: Text in this chapter is from "Treating Asthma with Bronchodilators," © 2009 The Cleveland Clinic Foundation, 9500 Euclid Avenue, Cleveland, OH 44195, www.clevelandclinic.org. Additional information is available from the Cleveland Clinic Health Information Center, (216) 444-3771, Toll Free: (800) 223-2273 extension 43771, or at http://www.clevelandclinic.org/health. Additional information about bronchodilators and asthma medicines is cited separately within the chapter.

- Albuterol (Proventil® HFA, Ventolin® HFA, AccuNeb®, ProAir®)

- Metaproterenol (Alupent®)

- Levalbuterol (Xopenex® HFA, Xopenex® nebulizer solution)

- Pirbuterol (Maxair®)

- Albuterol and ipratropium bromide combination (Combivent® metered dose inhaler; DuoNeb® solution)

Short-acting beta 2-agonists are also called "quick acting" or "rescue" medicines because they relieve asthma symptoms very quickly by opening the airways. These medications are the best for treating sudden and severe or new asthma symptoms. They work within 20 minutes and last four to six hours. They are also the medicines to use 15 to 20 minutes before exercise to prevent exercise-induced asthma symptoms. Albuterol is also available in oral form as pills or liquid. Overuse of short-acting beta 2-agonists is a sign of unstable asthma. If you need to use your short-acting beta 2-agonists more than twice per week, talk to your doctor about increasing the amounts of long-term control medicines you take, such as inhaled steroids and long-acting beta 2-agonists.

Beta 2-agonists—long-acting forms include:

- Salmeterol (Serevent®)

- Formoterol (Foradil®)

- Combination medications: salmeterol and fluticasone (Advair®); formoterol and budesonide (Symbicort®). These contain both the long-acting beta agonist and an inhaled corticosteroid. Symbicort® has recently been approved by the U.S. Food and Drug Administration (FDA).

☞ Remember!!

Note: The long-acting forms of beta 2-agonists are used to provide *control—not quick relief—*of asthma. These drugs may take longer to begin to work, but their benefits last 12 hours.

Source: © 2009 The Cleveland Clinic Foundation.

✔ Quick Tip
How are bronchodilators taken?

The best way to take a bronchodilator is to use an inhaler (or pump) with a spacer. A spacer is a plastic tube or bag that you attach to your pump to help get the medicine to your airways. One brand of bronchodilator for children over 12 years old is a dry powder inhaler and does not require the use of a spacer.

Side Effects: The side effects of bronchodilators may include rapid heartbeat, tremors, feeling anxious, and nausea. Serious side effects are rare, but may include chest pain, fast or irregular heart beat, severe headache or feeling dizzy, severe nausea, or vomiting. Call your doctor right away if you have any of these symptoms.

Source: From "Bronchodilators," reprinted with permission from the New York City Asthma Initiative, www.nyc.gov/health/asthma, New York City Department of Health and Mental Hygiene, March 2004.

Table 22.1. Quick Relief Medicines

Some Common Brand Names* Of Quick-Relief Medicines	Less Common Brand Names* of Quick-Relief Medicines
Albuterol (Albuterol is a generic name)	Alupent (Metaproterenol sulfate)
Proventil HFA (Albuterol)	Atrovent (Ipratropium bromide)
Proventil (Albuterol)	Brethine (Terbutaline sulfate)
Ventolin (Albuterol)	Maxair (Pirbuterol)
	Tornalate (Bitolterol)
	Volmax (Albuterol)
	Xopenex (Levalbuterol)

*Generic names in parentheses.

—Table reprinted with permission from "Bronchodilators," the New York City Asthma Initiative, www.nyc.gov/health/asthma, New York City Department of Health and Mental Hygiene, March 2004.

Salmeterol and formoterol are the only inhaled long-acting beta 2-agonists available. They are used twice a day to maintain open airways for long-term control and must be used in conjunction with an inhaled corticosteroid for the treatment of asthma. They have also been shown to be helpful in treating exercise-induced asthma. They are available in dry powder inhaler (DPI) form.

Side effects of beta 2-agonists include:

- nervous or shaky feeling;

- overexcitement or hyperactivity;

- increased heart rate;

- upset stomach (rare);

- trouble sleeping (rare).

Oral forms of beta 2-agonists (pills or syrups) tend to have more side effects because they are in higher doses and are absorbed throughout the bloodstream to get to the lungs. Inhaled forms are deposited directly in the lungs and therefore have fewer side effects.

Anticholinergic Drugs: There are two anticholinergic bronchodilators currently available: Ipratropium bromide (Atrovent® HFA), which is available as a metered dose inhaler and nebulizer solution; and tiotropium bromide (Spiriva®), which is a dry powder inhaler. Ipratropium is used four times per day, whereas tiotropium is used only once per day, as its action lasts for 24 hours. These are not quick relief medications but medications that can enhance the bronchodilator effect for certain asthmatics with difficult-to-control symptoms. Although not commonly used to treat asthma, they can be of benefit to some patients.

Side effects are minor; dry throat is the most common. If the medicine gets in your eyes, it might cause blurred vision for a short period of time.

Theophylline: Theophylline is another type of bronchodilator that is used to control asthma. Brand names include Uniphyl®, Theo-Dur®, Slo-bid®, and Theo-24®. Theophylline is available as a pill or as an intravenous (through the vein) drug. It is long-acting and prevents asthma attacks. Theophylline is used to treat difficult-to-control or severe asthma and must be taken daily.

Side effects include:

- nausea and/or vomiting;

- diarrhea;

- stomach ache;

- headache;

- rapid or irregular heartbeat;

- muscle cramps;

- jittery or nervous feeling;

- hyperactivity.

These side effects might be a warning of too much medicine. Your doctor will check your blood levels to make sure you're receiving the proper amount.

Always tell your doctors if you take theophylline for asthma because certain medicines—such as antibiotics containing erythromycin, or seizure or ulcer medicines—can interfere with the way theophylline works. Also, viral illnesses and cigarette smoking can change how your body responds to theophylline.

Chapter 23

What You Need To Know About Corticosteroids

In 1935, the Mayo Clinic reported a research breakthrough that would affect millions of lives. Doctors had isolated the hormone cortisone from the adrenal glands, the walnut sized glands sitting on top of the kidneys. Cortisone produced by the adrenal glands reduces inflammation in the body.

The Mayo Clinic physicians first used cortisone to treat people with severe rheumatoid arthritis. Improvements were so dramatic in soothing swollen joints that patients crippled from the disease were actually able to walk again.

Pharmaceutical companies have since produced corticosteroids medications that mimic the hormone cortisone. For people with asthma, corticosteroids literally can be lifesavers by preventing or reversing inflammation in the airways, making them less sensitive to triggers. The drugs, sometimes referred to as "preventive" or "long term control" medicines, work effectively to keep asthma episodes in check. They are not the same as anabolic steroids, which some athletes take illegally to build muscle mass.

Are Corticosteroids Safe?

Oral, or systemic, corticosteroids quickly help out-of-control asthma, but more than two weeks of daily use may sometimes lead to serious side effects. Inhaled corticosteroids are considered much safer for lengthier treatment. Unlike the oral forms that must travel throughout your body to reach your lungs, inhaled corticosteroids are delivered directly to the airways in small doses with less chance of reaching other parts of the body. The National Institutes of Health (NIH) calls inhaled corticosteroids "the most effective long-term therapy available for patients with persistent asthma. In general [they] are well tolerated and safe at the recommended dosages."

You have probably read or heard varying reports about the risks of corticosteroid use. The bottom line is that the relatively few side effects are usually balanced by the good they do for your asthma. Steroids are definitely safe when used in the lower dosage range. Problems generally arise with high doses over long periods of time. As consumers and patients, it's important to know what specific side effects may occur and how we can work with our physicians to control them and our asthma.

Localized Risks

Oral Candidiasis (Thrush): Only 10 percent to 30 percent of inhaled steroid doses actually reach the lungs. The remainder is left in the mouth or throat or is swallowed, sometimes resulting in thrush, a fungal infection that produces milky white lesions in the mouth. Clinical thrush is far less common in lower dosages and affects more adults than children.

Physicians recommend using a spacer or holding chamber with your inhaler and rinsing your mouth with water after each treatment to reduce the amount of the inhaled steroid deposited in the mouth and throat. If you develop thrush, your doctor may also prescribe a less frequent dose and/or topical or oral antifungal medication.

Dysphonia (Hoarseness): This condition is associated with increasing dosages of inhaled corticosteroids and vocal stress. Treatment may include using a spacer/holding chamber, less frequent dosing, and/or temporarily decreasing medication.

✤ It's A Fact!!

In a 1995 study of seven- to nine-year-olds treated daily with 400 mcg of beclomethasone for seven months, growth was significantly decreased in both boys and girls. There was no evidence of catch-up growth after a five month period without medication. Yet a 1994 study of inhaled beclomethasone found no significant adverse effects on achieving adult height.

The NIH advises physicians to carefully monitor a young patient's height and to "step down" therapy when possible. NIH notes that even high doses of inhaled corticosteroids with children experiencing severe, persistent asthma create less risk of delayed growth than treatment with oral systemic corticosteroids (pills or capsules).

Systemic Risks

Slowed Growth In Children: Some studies have shown that medium dose inhaled corticosteroids may affect a child's growth. It is not certain that this results in shorter stature in adulthood, but in general, the higher the dose, the greater the risk.

Osteoporosis (Bone Disease): In some people, high corticosteroid usage can reduce bone mineral density, leading to osteoporosis. Links have been found between steroid use and inhibiting bone formation, calcium absorption, and the production of sex hormones that help keep bones vital. Brief courses of systemic corticosteroids or low dose inhaled steroids are not dangerous, but inhaling 1500 micrograms of beclomethasone per day can lead to bone loss. The doses of other inhaled steroids, which may constitute a risk for osteoporosis, have not been studied.

Even if you need to take steroids for your asthma, you can take measures to protect yourself against osteoporosis. Here are some recommendations:

• Take the lowest dose possible and use inhaled steroids rather than oral preparations.

- Get about 1,500 mg of calcium daily through nutrition or supplements. Because vitamin D helps the body absorb calcium, it may help to take 800 international units (IU) daily of vitamin D.

- Receive replacement female hormone therapy unless prohibited for medical reasons. There are non-hormonal drugs available (bisphosphonates or calcitonin) that work similarly.

Disseminated Varicella (Chicken Pox): The U.S. Food and Drug Administration (FDA) reported that long-term or high-dose oral corticosteroid treatment might place people exposed to chicken pox or measles at increased risk of unusually severe infections or even death. That's because some doses suppress the immune system. "Children who are on immunosuppressant drugs

☞ **Remember!!**

Oral (Systemic) Corticosteroids

- Generally for short-term use
- Quickly controls persistent asthma
- Forms: pills, tablets, or liquid (for children)
- Medications: Methylprednisolone, Prednisolone, Prednisone

Inhaled Corticosteroids

- For long-term asthma prevention; suppress, control and reverse inflammation
- Forms: dry powder or aerosol
- Medications: Beclomethasone dipropionate, Budesonide, Flunisolide, Fluticasone propionate, Triamcinolone acetonide

are more susceptible to infections than healthy children," said the FDA. Yet, the NIH Guidelines said there is no evidence that recommended doses of inhaled corticosteroids suppress the immune system.

NIH advises that children who have not had chicken pox and periodically take oral corticosteroids should receive the Varicella vaccine after they've been steroid-free for at least one month. Kids who have finished a short course of prednisone may receive the vaccine immediately. For unimmunized adults and children who are exposed to chicken pox while being treated with immunosuppressive levels of steroids, there are immunoglobulin and acyclovir.

Table 23.1. What are Considered Low, Medium, And High Dosages?[1]

A = adult C = child

All dosages are daily, in micrograms (MCG).

Drug	Low	Medium	High
Beclomethasone	A 168–504	504–840	840+
dipropionate	C 84–336	336–672	672+
Budesonide	A 200–400	400–600	600+
Turbuhaler	C 100–200	200–400	400+
Flunisolide	A 500–1,000	1,000–2,000	2,000+
	C 500–750	1,000–1,250	1,250
Fluticasone	A 88–264	264–660	660+
	C 88–176	176–440	440+
Triamcinolone	A 400–1,000	1,000–2,000	2,000
acetonide	C 400–800	800–1,200	1,200

1. NIH Guidelines of the Diagnosis and Management of Asthma, April 1997.

Cataracts: The risk of cataracts in patients taking systemic corticosteroids has been well identified, but reports among those taking inhaled steroids are rare. In a notable exception, the *New England Journal of Medicine* published findings of a recent Australian study of inhaled corticosteroid users between the ages of 49 and 97. The authors concluded that the use of inhaled steroids is associated with an increased risk for development of cataracts. Patients taking moderate to high doses of inhaled corticosteroids especially should have regular eye exams.

Other Risks

The NIH Guidelines also list a few other rare but potential risks of high dose corticosteroid use. In some cases, oral steroid use has been linked with adrenal suppression, effects on glucose metabolism, and hypertension. Serious medical complications have also been recorded in people on high doses of oral steroids with tuberculosis.

None of the above risks have been reported with inhaled corticosteroids. However, their use in moderate to high doses has been found to contribute to thinning and bruising of the skin, especially among women.

Chapter 24

What You Need To Know About Cromolyn Sodium

Why is this medication prescribed?

Cromolyn is used to prevent the wheezing, shortness of breath, and troubled breathing caused by asthma. It also is used to prevent breathing difficulties (bronchospasm) during exercise. It works by preventing the release of substances that cause inflammation (swelling) in the air passages of the lungs.

This medication is sometimes prescribed for other uses; ask your doctor or pharmacist for more information.

How should this medicine be used?

Cromolyn comes as a solution and an aerosol to inhale by mouth. It is usually inhaled three or four times a day to prevent asthma attacks or within an hour before activities to prevent breathing difficulties caused by exercise.

Follow the directions on your prescription label carefully, and ask your doctor or pharmacist to explain any part you do not understand. Use cromolyn exactly as directed. Do not use more or less of it or use it more often than prescribed by your doctor.

About This Chapter: Text in this chapter is from "Cromolyn Sodium Oral Inhalation," © 2009 American Society of Health-System Pharmacists, Inc. All rights reserved. Any duplication in any form must be authorized by American Society of Health-System Pharmacists.

It may take up to four weeks for cromolyn to work. You should use it regularly for it to be effective. If your symptoms have not improved after four weeks, tell your doctor.

Cromolyn is used with a special inhaler. Before you use cromolyn inhalation for the first time, read the instructions for your device. Ask your doctor, pharmacist, or respiratory therapist to demonstrate the proper technique. Practice using your inhalation device while in his or her presence.

To use the inhaler, follow these steps:

- Shake the inhaler well

- Remove the protective cap

- Exhale (breathe out) as completely as possible through your nose while keeping your mouth shut

- Open Mouth Technique: Open your mouth wide, and place the open end of the mouthpiece about one or two inches from your mouth. Closed Mouth Technique: Place the open end of the mouthpiece well into your mouth, past your front teeth. Close your lips tightly around the mouthpiece.

- Take a slow, deep breath through the mouthpiece and, at the same time, press down on the container to spray the medication into your mouth. Be sure that the mist goes into your throat and is not blocked by your teeth or tongue. Adults giving the treatment to young children may hold the child's nose closed to be sure that the medication goes into the child's throat.

- Hold your breath for five to 10 seconds, remove the inhaler, and exhale slowly through your nose or mouth. If you take two puffs, wait two minutes and shake the inhaler well before taking the second puff.

- Replace the protective cap on the inhaler.

If you have difficulty getting the medication into your lungs, a spacer (a special device that attaches to the inhaler) may help; ask your doctor, pharmacist, or respiratory therapist.

What should I do if I forget a dose?

Use the missed dose as soon as you remember it. However, if it is almost time for the next dose, skip the missed dose and continue your regular dosing schedule. Do not use a double dose to make up for a missed one.

> ### ✔ Quick Tip
>
> ### What special precautions should I follow?
>
> Before using cromolyn:
>
> - tell your doctor and pharmacist if you are allergic to cromolyn or any other drugs;
> - tell your doctor and pharmacist what prescription and nonprescription medications you are taking, especially isoproterenol (Aerolone, Isuprel, others) and vitamins;
> - tell your doctor if you have or have ever had liver or kidney disease;
> - tell your doctor if you are pregnant, plan to become pregnant, or are breast-feeding. If you become pregnant while using cromolyn, call your doctor.

What side effects can this medication cause?

Cromolyn may cause side effects. Tell your doctor if any of these symptoms are severe or do not go away:

- Sore throat
- Bad taste in the mouth
- Stomach pain
- Cough
- Stuffy nose
- Itching or burning nasal passages
- Sneezing
- Headache

If you experience any of the following symptoms, call your doctor immediately:

- Wheezing
- Increased difficulty breathing
- Swelling of the tongue or throat

What storage conditions are needed for this medicine?

Keep this medication in the container it came in, tightly closed, and out of reach of children. Store it at room temperature and away from excess heat and moisture (not in the bathroom). Throw away any medication that is outdated or no longer needed. Talk to your pharmacist about the proper disposal of your medication. Avoid puncturing the aerosol container, and do not discard it in an incinerator or fire.

What other information should I know?

Keep all appointments with your doctor and the laboratory. Your doctor will order certain lab tests to check your response to cromolyn.

Do not use cromolyn to relieve an asthma attack that has already started; continue to use the medication prescribed for your acute attacks.

To relieve dry mouth or throat irritation caused by cromolyn inhalation, rinse your mouth with water, chew gum, or suck sugarless hard candy after each treatment.

Inhalation devices require regular cleaning. Once a week, remove the drug container from the plastic mouthpiece, wash the mouthpiece with warm tap water, and dry it thoroughly. Follow the written instructions for care of other inhalation devices.

Brand Names: Intal®

☞ Remember!!

Do not let anyone else use your medication. Ask your pharmacist any questions you have about refilling your prescription.

It is important for you to keep a written list of all of the prescription and nonprescription (over-the-counter) medicines you are taking, as well as any products such as vitamins, minerals, or other dietary supplements. You should bring this list with you each time you visit a doctor or if you are admitted to a hospital. It is also important information to carry with you in case of emergencies.

Chapter 25

What You Need To Know About Montelukast And Other Leukotriene Modifiers

Singulair (Montelukast)

The U.S. Food and Drug Administration (FDA) provided updated information to its March 2008 Early Communication. FDA is continuing to review clinical trial data to assess other neuropsychiatric events, (mood and behavioral adverse events) related to drugs that act through the leukotriene pathway (montelukast, zafirlukast, zileuton). As a result, FDA has not yet reached a definitive conclusion regarding the clinical trial data on mood and behavioral adverse events associated with montelukast, zafirlukast, and zileuton.

FDA informed health care professionals and patients of the Agency's investigation of the possible association between the use of Singulair and behavior/mood changes, suicidality (suicidal thinking and behavior) and suicide. Singulair is a leukotriene receptor antagonist used to treat asthma and the symptoms of allergic rhinitis, and to prevent exercise-induced asthma. Patients should not stop taking Singulair before talking to their doctor if they have questions about the new information. Health care professionals

About This Chapter: This chapter begins with information from U.S. Food and Drug Administration's MedWatch, March 2008 and January 2009. Other information from American Society of Health-System Pharmacists, Inc., the American Lung Association, CMPMedica Australia, and Family Allergy and Asthma is cited separately in the chapter.

and caregivers should monitor patients taking Singulair for suicidality (suicidal thinking and behavior) and changes in behavior and mood.

This early communication is in keeping with FDA's commitment to inform the public about its ongoing safety reviews of drugs. Due to the complexity of the analyses, FDA anticipates that it may take up to nine months to complete the ongoing evaluations. As soon as this review is complete, FDA will communicate the conclusions and recommendations to the public.

Montelukast

From "Montelukast," © 2009 American Society of Health-System Pharmacists, Inc. All rights reserved. Any duplication in any form must be authorized by American Society of Health-System Pharmacists.

Editorial Note: Although this material addresses parents, it is still helpful for teens to know.

Why is this medication prescribed?

Pending revision, the material in this section should be considered in light of more recently available information in the MedWatch notification at the beginning of this chapter.

Montelukast is used to prevent difficulty breathing, chest tightness, wheezing, and coughing caused by asthma. Montelukast is also used to prevent bronchospasm (breathing difficulties) during exercise. Montelukast is also used to treat the symptoms of seasonal (occurs only at certain times of the year), and perennial (occurs all year round) allergic rhinitis (a condition associated with sneezing and stuffy, runny or itchy nose). Montelukast is in a class of medications called leukotriene receptor antagonists (LTRAs). It works by blocking the action of substances in the body that cause the symptoms of asthma and allergic rhinitis.

How should this medicine be used?

Montelukast comes as a tablet, a chewable tablet, and granules to take by mouth. Montelukast is usually taken once a day with or without food. When montelukast is used to treat asthma, it should be taken in the evening. When montelukast is used to prevent breathing difficulties during exercise, it should be taken at least two hours before exercise. If you are taking montelukast once a day on a regular basis, you should not take an additional dose before exercising. When montelukast is used to treat allergic rhinitis, it may be taken at any time of day. Take montelukast at around the same time every day. Follow the directions on your prescription label carefully, and ask your doctor or pharmacist to explain any part you do not understand. Take montelukast exactly as directed. Do not take more or less of it or take it more often than prescribed by your doctor.

If you are giving the granules to your child, you should not open the foil pouch until your child is ready to take the medication. There are several ways that you can give the granules to your child, so choose the one that works best for you and your child. You may pour all of the granules directly from the packet into your child's mouth to be swallowed immediately. You may also pour the entire packet of granules onto a clean spoon and place the spoonful of medication in your child's mouth. If you prefer, you may mix the entire packet of granules in one teaspoon of cold or room temperature baby formula, breast milk, applesauce, soft carrots, ice cream, or rice. You should not mix the granules with any other foods or liquids, but your child may drink any liquid right after he or she takes the granules. If you mix the granules with one of the allowed foods or drinks, use the mixtures within 15 minutes. Do not store unused mixtures of food, formula, or breast milk and the medication.

Do not use montelukast to treat a sudden attack of asthma symptoms. Your doctor will prescribe a short-acting inhaler to use during attacks. Talk to your doctor about how to treat symptoms of a sudden asthma attack. If your asthma symptoms get worse or if you have asthma attacks more often, be sure to call your doctor.

If you are taking montelukast to treat asthma, continue to take or use all other medications that your doctor has prescribed to treat your asthma. Do not stop taking any of your medications or change the doses of any of your medications unless your doctor tells you that you should. If your asthma is made worse by aspirin, do not take aspirin or other non-steroidal anti-inflammatory drugs (NSAIDs) during your treatment with montelukast.

Other Uses For This Medicine: This medication may be prescribed for other uses; ask your doctor or pharmacist for more information.

What special precautions should I follow?

Pending revision, the material in this section should be considered in light of more recently available information in the MedWatch notification at the beginning of this chapter.

Before taking montelukast:

- tell your doctor and pharmacist if you are allergic to montelukast or any other medications;

- tell your doctor and pharmacist what prescription and nonprescription medications, vitamins, nutritional supplements, and herbal products you are taking or plan to take. Be sure to mention phenobarbital and rifampin (Rifadin, Rimactane). Your doctor may need to change the doses of your medications or monitor you more carefully for side effects.

- tell your doctor if you have or have ever had liver disease;

- tell your doctor if you are pregnant, plan to become pregnant, or are breast feeding. If you become pregnant while taking montelukast, call your doctor.

- if you have phenylketonuria (PKU, an inherited condition in which a special diet must be followed to prevent mental retardation), you should know that the chewable tablets contain aspartame that forms phenylalanine.

What special dietary instructions should I follow?

Unless your doctor tells you otherwise, continue your normal diet.

What should I do if I forget a dose?

Skip the missed dose and continue your regular dosing schedule. Do not take a double dose to make up for a missed one. Do not take more than one dose of montelukast in a 24 hour period.

☞ Remember!!

Montelukast controls the symptoms of asthma and allergic rhinitis but does not cure these conditions. Continue to take montelukast even if you feel well. Do not stop taking montelukast without talking to your doctor. Ask your pharmacist or doctor for a copy of the manufacturer's information for the patient.

Source: © 2009 American Society of Health-System Pharmacists, Inc.

What side effects can this medication cause?

Pending revision, the material in this chapter should be considered in light of more recently available information in the MedWatch notification at the beginning of this chapter.

Montelukast may cause side effects. Tell your doctor if any of these symptoms are severe or do not go away:

• Headache

• Dizziness

• Heartburn

• Stomach pain

• Tiredness

Some side effects can be serious. If you experience any of the following symptoms, call your doctor immediately:

• Difficulty breathing or swallowing

• Swelling of the face, throat, tongue, lips, eyes, hands, feet, ankles, or lower legs

• Hoarseness

• Itching

- Rash

- Hives

- Fever

- Flu-like symptoms

- Pins and needles or numbness in the arms or legs

- Pain and swelling of the sinuses

Montelukast may cause other side effects. Call your doctor if you have any unusual problems while you are taking this medication.

If you experience a serious side effect, you or your doctor may send a report to the Food and Drug Administration's (FDA) MedWatch Adverse Event Reporting program online at http://www .fda.gov/MedWatch/index.html or by phone (800) 332-1088.

> **✔ Quick Tip**
> **In Case Of**
> **Emergency Or Overdose**
>
> In case of overdose, call your local poison control center at (800) 222-1222. If the victim has collapsed or is not breathing, call local emergency services at 911.
>
> Symptoms of overdose may include:
>
> - stomach pain;
> - sleepiness
> - thirst
> - headache
> - vomiting
> - restlessness or agitation
>
> Source: © 2009 American Society of Health-System Pharmacists, Inc.

What storage conditions are needed for this medicine?

Keep this medication in the container it came in, tightly closed, and out of reach of children. Store it at room temperature and away from excess heat and moisture (not in the bathroom). Throw away any medication that is outdated or no longer needed. Talk to your pharmacist about the proper disposal of your medication.

What other information should I know?

Pending revision, the material in this section should be considered in light of more recently available information in the MedWatch notification at the beginning of this chapter. Keep all appointments with your doctor. Do not let anyone else take your medication. Ask your pharmacist any questions you have about refilling your prescription.

It is important for you to keep a written list of all of the prescription and nonprescription (over-the-counter) medicines you are taking, as well as any products such as vitamins, minerals, or other dietary supplements. You should bring this list with you each time you visit a doctor or if you are admitted to a hospital. It is also important information to carry with you in case of emergencies.

Brand Names: Singulair®

American Lung Association Study Finds No Evidence Of Depression Or Suicide Linked To Asthma And Allergy Drug Montelukast

Excerpted from "American Lung Association Study Finds No Evidence of Depression or Suicide Linked to Asthma and Allergy Drug Montelukast," © 2009 American Lung Association. Reprinted with permission. For more information about the American Lung Association or to support the work it does, call 800-LUNG-USA (800-586-4872) or log on to www.LungUSA.org.

There has been recent concern that suicide may be a complication of montelukast (Singulair) therapy. Montelukast is a Food and Drug Administration (FDA) approved oral drug that has been prescribed for more than a decade for the treatment of asthma and seasonal allergy symptoms. An independent study sponsored by the American Lung Association has found no evidence of depression or suicide linked to Montelukast.

American Lung Association researchers Janet Holbrook, PhD, MPH and Raida Harik-Khan, PhD have re-analyzed data from patients who had participated in past clinical trials involving montelukast conducted by the Association's Asthma Clinical Research Centers (ACRC) Network to identify any signals that might suggest a link between montelukast and its effect on emotional well-being. They report their findings in an upcoming issue of the *Journal of Allergy and Clinical Immunology*.

"Discovering adverse effects of a drug after it is on the market can be very difficult, because the data are usually gathered from single events reported by doctors, which makes it is challenging to differentiate actual side effects from events unrelated to the drug," said Norman Edelman, MD American Lung Association Chief Medical Officer. "The value of this 'look back' study is that the investigators were able to compare a large group of patients given montelukast with those given a placebo making a firm scientific conclusion possible."

Holbrook and Harik-Khan reviewed quality of life and emotional well being data collected from patients in three American Lung Association ACRC Network clinical trials that had used montelukast as one of their treatments. Of the 1,352 patients who participated in the double-blind, controlled studies, 569 of these patients had been randomly assigned to take montelukast. The researchers analyzed these patients' data and found no evidence of any deterioration of emotional well being in either the adults or the children who received montelukast. On the contrary, the research team found a positive effect on emotional outlook when comparing patients taking montelukast to those receiving placebo.

While the findings of this study are reassuring and produced no evidence to support the recent publicity regarding a link between montelukast and depression or suicide, the authors do not dismiss the possibility that there could be other unrecognized adverse reactions to montelukast.

Source: Reprinted with permission. © 2009 American Lung Association.

Leukotriene Receptor Antagonists For Asthma Treatment

From "Leukotriene Receptor Antagonists for Asthma Treatment," reprinted with permission from www.mydr.com.au © 2007 CMPMedica Australia.

In the past few years, a class of medicines known as leukotriene receptor antagonists has been developed for the treatment of asthma.

Leukotriene receptor antagonists, such as montelukast sodium (e.g., Singulair tablets) or zafirlukast (e.g., Accolate tablets), are not used to treat an acute attack of asthma. They are preventers and come in tablet form. Leukotriene receptor antagonists should be taken daily, as prescribed.

Leukotriene receptor antagonists treat asthma via a totally different pathway to other available medicines. They work by blocking substances in your lungs called leukotrienes, which cause narrowing and swelling of the airways in asthma.

Montelukast and zafirlukast are used to help prevent asthma symptoms. As they come in tablet form, leukotriene receptor antagonists are especially useful in children or adults who cannot use puffers. Montelukast can be taken by children older than two and by adults, while zafirlukast can be taken only by those 12 years old or older.

☞ Remember!!
Types Of Leukotriene Modifiers

Montelukast (Singulair®) is the only once-a-day leukotriene modifier and is taken orally. Bronchodilator effects may begin within two hours, but the preventive anti-inflammatory effects will not begin for up to one week. Side effects may include headache, fatigue, fever, intestinal symptoms, laryngitis, and/or pharyngitis.

Zafirlukast (Accolate®) is taken orally, and generally is prescribed twice a day. Zafirlukast (Accolate®) should be taken on an empty stomach, one hour *before* or two hours *after* a meal. As with Montelukast (Singulair®), bronchodilator effects may begin within two hours, but preventive effects will not begin for up to one week. Side effects may include headache, dizziness, infection, nausea, vomiting, or diarrhea.

Zileuton (ZyfloCR®) is taken orally, two times a day. Be sure you do not decrease dosage on your own without consulting your physician, even if you are feeling better. Side effects may include headache, nausea, abdominal pain, or indigestion. Some patients may develop abnormal liver function while on this medication. If you have a known liver problem, you should avoid using Zileuton (ZyfloCR®). Liver function will be monitored if this medication is prescribed.

Source: From "Asthma Classification," © 2009 Family Allergy and Asthma (www.familyallergy.com). All rights reserved. Reprinted with permission.

Your doctor can advise if a leukotriene receptor antagonist is suitable for you or your child. Tell your doctor if you are pregnant or planning to become pregnant, or if you are breast feeding or planning to do so, as they may wish to prescribe a different medicine for you.

The most common side effects of leukotriene receptor antagonists are headache and gastrointestinal upsets.

Chapter 26

What You Need To Know About Theophylline

Theophylline: Revisiting An Old Asthma Treatment

In this section we discuss the use of theophylline for asthma both in the past and present. While this medication has fallen out of favor as a first line medication in the treatment of asthma, it should not be overlooked as an option for many patients with asthma.

Theophylline In The Past And Present

Theophylline is a drug that has been in use for asthma since the 1950s. Structurally related to caffeine, it was first isolated from tea leaves in the late 19th century. Current drug preparations are synthesized in the laboratory.

In the early days of drug treatment for asthma, there were limited treatments—most of the drugs had significant side effects because they didn't directly target the breathing tubes of individuals with asthma. The airways

About This Chapter: This chapter begins with "Theophylline: Revisiting An Old Asthma Treatment" written by Dr. Fred Little for The HealthCentral Network, Inc. and first published on HealthCentral's asthma website www.MyAsthmaCentral.com, March 2, 2008. Copyright © 2008 The HealthCentral Network, Inc. All Rights Reserved. Additional information from the American Lung Association and the American Society of Health-System Pharmacists, Inc. is cited separately in the chapter.

of people with asthma could be relaxed but at a cost of side effects on other parts of the body:

- Steroids weakened bones and the immune system and caused weight gain

- Epinephrine was short acting and strained the heart

Theophylline was recognized as a drug that could loosen tight airways, but for this effect, blood levels needed to be at a point that caused jitteriness and upset stomach (similar to the effects from an "overdose" of caffeine). Because there were few alternatives, most patients with chronic asthma that caused daily symptoms between the 1960s and 1980s were taking some preparation of theophylline.

During the 1980s, there were several developments in asthma treatments that changed the lives of asthma sufferers and decreased the use of theophylline. More selective bronchodilators (drugs that relax the breathing tubes or "airways") with fewer side effects were discovered, such as albuterol. Steroids could be given through an inhaler to deliver medication directly to the lungs without having to go through the rest of the body, thus avoiding side effects of steroids given in pill form or by injection.

Because of these powerful new treatments, as well as the modest benefits of theophylline and its side effects, theophylline fell out of favor. In the late 1990s, theophylline was relegated to second or third line status in the treatment of chronic asthma.

New Findings About Theophylline

The main limitations to the use of theophylline in the past have been its side effects and the fact that it is a relatively weak bronchodilator compared to albuterol and related inhaled medicines. But recent research has shown that there may be newer, underappreciated effects of theophylline. Theophylline can improve breathing in other ways, such as strengthening the diaphragm, the main muscle that we use to bring air into our lungs. In addition, theophylline has been shown to have so-called 'anti-inflammatory' effects on the airways. This effect directly combats the abnormal inflammation in the airways of asthmatics. Most importantly, this effect is found at levels in the blood well below that which causes the common side effects seen in most people.

While theophylline is still not a reasonable choice as a *sole* agent in asthma treatment, its use is being reevaluated as an option to *add on* to existing medications in an individual whose asthma is not optimally controlled.

Closing Thoughts

While there are many newer medications for the treatment of chronic asthma with few side effects, some patients may benefit from the addition of theophylline to their current medication regimen. With new treatment guidelines, there are fewer side effects as the target level in the blood is lower than in past times. Whether theophylline is an option for your asthma treatment should be discussed with your doctor.

Theophylline

Why is this medication prescribed?

Theophylline is used to prevent and treat wheezing, shortness of breath, and difficulty breathing caused by asthma, chronic bronchitis, emphysema, and other lung diseases. It relaxes and opens air passages in the lungs, making it easier to breathe.

This medication is sometimes prescribed for other uses; ask your doctor or pharmacist for more information.

How should this medicine be used?

Theophylline comes as a tablet, capsule, solution, and syrup to take by mouth. It usually is taken every 6, 8, 12, or 24 hours. Follow the directions on your prescription label carefully, and ask your doctor or pharmacist to explain any part you do not understand. Take theophylline exactly as directed. Do not take more or less of it or take it more often than prescribed by your doctor.

Take this medication with a full glass of water on an empty stomach, at least one hour before or two hours after a meal. Do not chew or crush the

♣ **It's A Fact!!**

Theophylline is a bronchodilator, meaning that it relieves the constriction in your airways. It also increases the ability of the diaphragm to contract and improves clearance of mucus from the airways. Theophylline may improve the benefits of other asthma medications, so it is often prescribed as part of an overall asthma action plan.

Viral upper respiratory infections with fever, high carbohydrate diets, liver failure, birth control pills, and alcoholic beverages may increase theophylline levels. Cigarettes, high protein diets, and charcoal-broiled foods can lower theophylline levels. Theophylline has the potential for many side effects and interactions with other drugs, so be sure to discuss all medications, prescribed and over-the-counter, you are taking with your doctor. Lifestyle and diet should also be discussed to be sure that theophylline is taken safely and effectively.

Theophylline is generally taken orally, but may be given intravenously. Current brands of theophylline include:

- Slo-bid®;
- Theophylline®;
- Theo-24®;
- Uni-Dur®;
- Uniphyl®.

Possible side effects may include headache, hyperactivity, insomnia, upset stomach, irritation of ulcers, or gastroesophageal reflux (heartburn). Elderly males with prostate problems may have difficulty in urination and will be monitored.

Source: From "Asthma Classification," © 2009 Family Allergy and Asthma (www.familyallergy.com). All rights reserved. Reprinted with permission.

extended-release (long-acting) tablets; swallow them whole. Extended-release capsules (e.g., Theo-Dur Sprinkles) may be swallowed whole or opened and the contents mixed with soft food and swallowed without chewing.

Theophylline controls symptoms of asthma and other lung diseases but does not cure them. Continue to take theophylline even if you feel well. Do not stop taking theophylline without talking to your doctor.

Other Uses For This Medicine: Theophylline is sometimes used to treat breathing problems in premature infants. Talk to your doctor about the possible risks of using this drug for your baby's condition.

What special precautions should I follow?

Before taking theophylline:

- Tell your doctor and pharmacist if you are allergic to theophylline or any other drugs.

- Tell your doctor and pharmacist what prescription medications you are taking, especially allopurinol (Zyloprim), azithromycin (Zithromax), carbamazepine (Tegretol), cimetidine (Tagamet), ciprofloxacin (Cipro), clarithromycin (Biaxin), diuretics ('water pills'), erythromycin, lithium (Eskalith, Lithobid), oral contraceptives, phenytoin (Dilantin), prednisone (Deltasone), propranolol (Inderal), rifampin (Rifadin), tetracycline (Sumycin), and other medications for infections or heart disease.

- Tell your doctor and pharmacist what nonprescription medications and vitamins you are taking, including ephedrine, epinephrine, phenylephrine, phenylpropanolamine, or pseudoephedrine. Many nonprescription products contain these drugs (e.g., diet pills and medications for colds and asthma), so check labels carefully. Do not take these medications without talking to your doctor; they can increase the side effects of theophylline.

- Tell your doctor if you have or have ever had seizures, ulcers, heart disease, an overactive or underactive thyroid gland, high blood pressure, or liver disease or if you have a history of alcohol abuse.

- Tell your doctor if you are pregnant, plan to become pregnant, or are breast feeding. If you become pregnant while taking theophylline, call your doctor.

- Tell your doctor if you use tobacco products. Cigarette smoking may decrease the effectiveness of theophylline.

What special dietary instructions should I follow?

Drinking or eating foods high in caffeine, like coffee, tea, cocoa, and chocolate, may increase the side effects caused by theophylline. Avoid large amounts of these substances while you are taking theophylline.

What should I do if I forget a dose?

Take the missed dose as soon as you remember it. However, if it is almost time for the next dose, skip the missed dose and continue your regular dosing schedule. Do not take a double dose to make up for a missed one. If you become severely short of breath, call your doctor.

What storage conditions are needed for this medicine?

Keep this medication in the container it came in, tightly closed, and out of reach of children. Store it at room temperature and away from excess heat and moisture (not in the bathroom). Throw away any medication that is outdated or no longer needed. Talk to your pharmacist about the proper disposal of your medication.

What other information should I know?

Keep all appointments with your doctor and the laboratory. Your doctor will order certain lab tests to check your response to theophylline.

Do not change from one brand of theophylline to another without talking to your doctor.

☞ Remember!! What side effects can this medication cause?

Theophylline may cause side effects. Tell your doctor if any of these symptoms are severe or do not go away:

- Upset stomach

- Stomach pain

- Diarrhea

- Headache

- Restlessness

- Insomnia

- Irritability

If you experience any of the following symptoms, call your doctor immediately:

- Vomiting

- Increased or rapid heart rate

- Irregular heartbeat

- Seizures

- Skin rash

If you experience a serious side effect, you or your doctor may send a report to the Food and Drug Administration's (FDA) MedWatch Adverse Event Reporting program online at http://www.fda.gov/MedWatch/index.html or by phone (800) 332-1088.

Source: © 2009 American Society of Health-System Pharmacists, Inc.

Do not let anyone else take your medication. Ask your pharmacist any questions you have about refilling your prescription.

It is important for you to keep a written list of all of the prescription and nonprescription (over-the-counter) medicines you are taking, as well as any products such as vitamins, minerals, or other dietary supplements. You should bring this list with you each time you visit a doctor or if you are admitted to a hospital. It is also important information to carry with you in case of emergencies.

Brand names: Bronkodyl®, Elixophyllin®, Slo-bid®, Slo-Phyllin®, Theo-24®, Theo-Dur®, Theolair®, Uniphyl®.

Asthma Treatment Options Clarified, American Lung Association Reports

From "Asthma Treatment Options Clarified, American Lung Association Reports," © 2009 American Lung Association. Reprinted with permission. For more information about the American Lung Association or to support the work it does, call 800-LUNG-USA (800-586-4872) or log on to www.LungUSA.org.

Results Of Asthma Clinical Research Centers Study Examined Poorly Controlled Asthma

A nationwide, multi-center clinical trial of the American Lung Association's Asthma Clinical Research Centers (ACRC) has found that neither low-dose theophylline nor montelukast improve asthma control in

✔ Quick Tip
In Case Of Emergency/Overdose

In case of overdose, call your local poison control center at (800) 222-1222. If the victim has collapsed or is not breathing, call local emergency services at 911.

Source: © 2009 American Society of Health-System Pharmacists, Inc.

people who were using just a short acting inhaled bronchodilator, but that low-dose theophylline is beneficial in those patients who had not been prescribed inhaled corticosteroids.

"Our study confirms that low-dose theophylline is a useful alternative in those patients who are not able or willing to take inhaled corticosteroids," said Norman H. Edelman, MD, American Lung Association Chief Medical Officer. "Inhaled corticosteroids have become a mainstay of asthma treatment. The results of our research offer greater data for physicians treating patients who cannot or will not use inhaled corticosteroids. And true to the goals of our Asthma Clinical Research Centers program, this is information that physicians can immediately use to help manage their patients' asthma," said Dr. Edelman.

Study results, "Clinical Trial of Low-Dose Theophylline and Montelukast in Patients with Poorly Controlled Asthma," were published in the February [2009] issue of the *American Journal of Respiratory and Clinical Care Medicine.*

Asthma symptoms, quality of life, and asthma control were consistent between both the treatment and control groups, although patients who took theophylline experienced more nausea and nervousness than those taking the placebo.

Source: The above information reprinted with permission. © 2009 American Lung Association.

Chapter 27

Inhaled Steroids

Inhaled steroids, also called inhaled corticosteroids, are considered to be the most effective medications for controlling asthma when taken regularly. They work continuously to reduce swelling of the airways.

Inhaled steroids include:

- Budesonide (Pulmicort®);

- Fluticasone (Flovent®);

- Ciclesonide (Alvesco®);

- Beclomethasone dipropionate (QVAR®).

If you're taking inhaled steroids and start to feel better, do not stop taking them. You must take them regularly and for as long as your doctor advises if you want to properly control your asthma.

The dose of the corticosteroid inhaler is in micrograms, which is one millionth of a gram. Corticosteroids in a tablet form (e.g., Prednisone) are in grams, a much higher dose than in the inhaler. Wherever possible, the least amount of

About This Chapter: Text in this chapter is from "Inhaled Steroids," and "All About Inhaled Steroids," reprinted with permission from the Asthma Society of Canada, © 2009. All rights reserved. For additional information about asthma, visit http://www.asthma.ca. Additional information from Permanente Medical Group is cited separately in the chapter.

medication is used to maintain asthma control. Corticosteroid tablets or liquid are used when a larger dose is needed to get the asthma under control.

Taking inhaled steroids can have a few side effects, but they are generally not serious. They include:

✤ **It's A Fact!!**

Inhaled corticosteroids are the most effective prescribed medication for most patients with asthma. Inhaled corticosteroids at the dose they are currently recommending for asthma have **not** been shown to cause weak bones, growth suppression, weight gain, and cataracts.

Source: © 2009 Asthma Society of Canada.

• hoarse voice;

• sore throat;

• mild throat infection (thrush).

You can minimize these side effects by rinsing your mouth after every dose of inhaled steroids and by using a spacer device with a pressurized metered-dose inhaler (pMDI).

There are a number of misconceptions about inhaled corticosteroids. For example, some people mistakenly believe that they are the same as the anabolic steroids that are sometimes abused by athletes. You can find out the truth about inhaled steroids in the next section.

All About Inhaled Steroids

Doctors generally prescribe inhaled corticosteroids over oral (tablet or liquid) corticosteroids, because the inhaled medication is more targeted. In other words, when it's inhaled, medication goes directly into the lungs where it's needed. Unlike oral medicines, inhaled steroids do not have to pass through other parts of the body where they're not needed, and as a result are less likely to cause unwanted side effects.

If you are using a pressurized MDI (pMDI) inhaled steroid, then doctors recommend the use of a spacer device, especially for children. A spacer slows down the delivery of the aerosol droplets that carry the medicine, making delivery even better targeted to get into the airways. Remember, spacers should not be used with dry-powered devices such as the DISKUS® or Turbuhaler®.

What are steroids?

Some athletes misuse anabolic steroids to build muscle. Corticosteroids are the steroids used to treat asthma. Corticosteroids do not build muscle or enhance performance. Corticosteroids are hormones that your body naturally produces. When your doctor prescribes an inhaled corticosteroid, he is giving a very small amount of this same hormone, to reduce the inflammation in the airways.

Will corticosteroids used to treat asthma cause dangerous side effects?

The corticosteroids that are inhaled to treat asthma today are considered safe. This is because the medicine, which is breathed in through a puffer, goes directly into the lungs where it reduces inflammation in the airways. A steroid tablet that is swallowed has more side effects because a large amount goes into the blood stream and is carried to other parts of the body. Side effects from inhaled corticosteroids are minor when the proper amount is taken. A few people get a cough, hoarseness or husky voice, sore throat or thrush (a yeast infection). Patients can protect against these discomforts by rinsing their mouth, gargling with water and spitting out, to remove any medicine left in the mouth.

Are inhaled corticosteroids reserved for people with severe asthma?

No. Inhaled corticosteroids are used in mild to moderate asthma as well as in more severe cases. Canada's Asthma Control Guidelines, developed by Canada's leading asthma doctors, recommend the use of inhaled corticosteroids to reduce airway inflammation and get symptoms under control.

How do I know that inhaled corticosteroids won't cause health problems in the longer term?

As with any medicine, doctors and patients must weigh the possible risks of taking medicine against the effects of not taking the medicine to decide what is best. Low amounts of inhaled steroids are generally considered to be the best option and are used by many people for asthma control.

I do not feel comfortable taking inhaled steroids every day. Can I stop?

When your asthma is under control talk to your doctor about adjusting the dose of your medications. Do not stop taking your controller medications. If you do, the airway inflammation may return.

About Inhaled Steroids

From "About Inhaled Steroids," reprinted with permission from The Permanente Medical Group, Inc., © 2008.

[Editor's Note: Although the following material is written to parents, it is still helpful for teens to know.]

What are inhaled steroids?

Inhaled steroids are medicines that reduce swelling in the airways of the lungs. If you or your child has asthma, your doctor may prescribe inhaled steroids for use every day to prevent asthma flare-ups. You or your child breathes inhaled steroids (such as QVAR, Asmanex, Flovent or Pulmicort) into the lungs. They are similar to a hormone called "cortisone" that our bodies make naturally.

✔ Quick Tip
Tips To Prevent Or Reduce The Risk Of ...

Yeast Infection In Your Mouth (Thrush)
- Always use your inhaler with a spacer. Check with your doctor about the correct spacer for you or your child.
- Always rinse out your mouth (rinse and spit) after you take the medicine.
- Use your inhaler before you brush your teeth.

Cough, Hoarseness, Or Husky Voice
- Rinse your mouth, gargling with water and spitting out, to remove any medicine left in your mouth.

Taking inhaled steroids has fewer risks than not controlling your asthma!

Source: © 2008 The Permanente Medical Group, Inc.[Editor's Note: Although this material is written to parents, it is still helpful for teens to know.]

Inhaled steroids help the airways to become less sensitive to the things that "trigger" asthma, so they make breathing easier. Since inhaled steroids do not work right away, it may take some time for you or your child to feel the benefits.

Are inhaled steroids the same as steroids body builders use?

No. Some body builders may use testosterone, a type of "anabolic" hormone to "bulk up." Testosterone is very different from the inhaled steroid you or your child uses to control asthma. The inhaled steroids do not build muscle or improve performance. In fact, using inhaled steroids allows athletes with asthma to breathe easier and to participate fully in sports.

What about side effects?

Inhaled steroids have few side effects. They are generally safe when used in the low doses that are usually prescribed. There can be a higher risk of side effects if you or your child uses high doses of inhaled steroids.

How can I use the least amount of inhaled steroids to control my or my child's asthma?

One way to reduce the amount of inhaled steroid you or your child takes is to control and avoid asthma triggers. You may be able to use less medicine if you reduce or avoid your asthma triggers (such as indoor pets, dust mites, cockroaches, pollen, cigarette and fireplace smoke, or strong odors). Managing your asthma with the least amount of medicine needed can help reduce any side effects you may have. If you are on a high dose of inhaled steroids ask your doctor if you might be able to take another medication that can help lower the dose you need.

Is there an increased risk of cataracts and glaucoma with inhaled steroids?

Some recent studies have suggested that patients over 65 on high doses of inhaled steroids may have a greater risk of getting cataracts and glaucoma. Patients using lower doses of inhaled steroids do not appear to be at higher risk of glaucoma. If you are taking high doses of inhaled steroids, check with your doctor, especially if you have glaucoma or one of these risk factors for glaucoma:

- diabetes mellitus (high sugar in your blood);

- extreme nearsightedness;

- a blood relative with glaucoma.

Your doctor may refer you to have your eyes checked by an eye specialist.

Is there an increased risk of osteoporosis (thinning of the bones) with inhaled steroids?

This issue is still being studied and we don't have all the answers yet. Some studies suggest that taking inhaled steroids can increase the risk of osteoporosis. Anyone can decrease their chances of osteoporosis (whether or not you are taking inhaled steroids) with regular physical activity. Taking a calcium supplement (1,000–1,500 mg/day) and vitamin D (400 units/day, the dose in most multiple vitamins) may help prevent bone thinning. If you have questions about any of these preventive measures, check with your doctor.

Will inhaled steroids affect my child's growth?

During the first year using inhaled steroids a child's growth may be slightly affected. On average, studies show that it can slow growth by a half inch. After the first year of treatment, the child's growth rate "catches up" and returns to normal. When used regularly, inhaled steroids are the best medicines to control asthma. Asthma that is not controlled causes growth to slow as well. Be sure to work with your child's doctor to find the lowest dose of inhaled steroids to keep asthma well-controlled.

Can I become addicted to inhaled steroids?

No. Inhaled steroids are not addictive. However, you must use them regularly to get the full benefit.

Are inhaled steroids safe to use during pregnancy?

Inhaled steroids are generally safe to use during pregnancy in the usual recommended doses. Be sure to let your doctor know right away if you are pregnant. He or she may need to change your inhaled steroid to a different brand.

Chapter 28

Do Inhaled Steroids Stunt Your Growth?

Teens may worry whether medication used to treat their asthma will make them shorter as adults. A great deal of research has been performed on this subject; this chapter will look at the basis of these concerns, and describe what the evidence tells us.

What are corticosteroids, and why do we give them to asthmatics?

Corticosteroids are a group of hormones that have widespread effects in the human body. Cortisol is produced in the adrenal glands. Among many other functions, it influences immune function, metabolism, blood pressure, and bone growth. A number of synthetic hormones with effects similar to cortisol have been developed to treat a variety of disease conditions. Commonly used corticosteroids include prednisone, prednisolone, triamcinolone, beclomethasone, budesonide, and fluticasone.

Asthma is a disease where chronic airway inflammation is present throughout the lungs. This inflammation leads to airway narrowing through muscle spasm, swelling, and excess mucus production. Reducing the inflammation is essential to treating asthma.

About This Chapter: Text in this chapter was written for Omnigraphics by David A. Cooke, MD, FACP. Dr. Cooke is board-certified in Internal Medicine and practices in Ann Arbor, Michigan. © 2004, Omnigraphics, Inc. Reviewed in 2009.

Corticosteroids have potent anti-inflammatory effects. In asthma, they are used to reduce airway swelling and spasm and stop excess mucus production. This results in less wheezing, less shortness of breath, and increased ability to participate in everyday activities.

Because the inflammation in asthma is mainly confined to the lungs, corticosteroids are most often given as an inhaled mist or powder. This delivers the medication directly to where it is needed.

✎ What's It Mean?

Adrenal Glands: A pair of yellow, triangle-shaped glands; one sits on top of each kidney. They produce many different important hormones.

Adult Height: How tall you are when you stop growing. Most teens stop growing between age fifteen and nineteen; a few may stop sooner or grow longer.

Bronchodilators: Medications that open airways and relieve shortness of breath. Albuterol is one commonly used bronchodilator medication. Most give quick relief, but they don't treat the inflammation that causes asthma.

Corticosteroids: Hormones made in the human body that reduce inflammation. Many are used as medications.

Growth Velocity: How quickly a person is growing. For example, growing one inch taller per year.

Inflammation: Irritated and swollen tissue, packed with angry white blood cells.

Leukotriene Modifiers: Medications which reduce inflammation in a different way than corticosteroids or mast cell stabilizers. Montelukast, Zafirlukast, and Zileuton are the most commonly used forms. They are also less powerful than corticosteroids, but may be helpful when corticosteroids alone don't stop asthma symptoms.

Mast Cell Stabilizers: Medications to prevent certain cells from releasing hormones that cause more inflammation. Cromolyn and nedocromil are the most commonly used mast cell stabilizers. They have anti-inflammatory effects, but are weaker medications than corticosteroids.

Methylxanthines: An older type of asthma medication that helps open airways. Theophylline is an example. They do not treat inflammation. They are not used often today because of side effects and tricky dosing.

Why are there concerns about corticosteroids use in children and teens?

While corticosteroids reduce inflammation, they have many other effects. When given in high doses, corticosteroids reduce bone growth. In growing children and teens, this might lead to slowed growth and shorter heights as adults.

There is little question that these negative effects of corticosteroids are seen when they are given in high doses for months or years by oral or intravenous routes. Inhaled corticosteroids are given in much lower doses, and they are delivered mainly to the lungs. Some of the inhaled medication is absorbed into the bloodstream from the lungs, however, and could have effects elsewhere in the body.

If corticosteroids might have these risks, why don't we use other kinds of medications?

A number of medications have been developed for treatment of asthma. These include bronchodilators (such as albuterol), mast cell stabilizers (such as cromolyn), leukotriene modifiers (such as montelukast), and methylxanthines (such as theophylline). Each of these medication types have their roles in asthma therapy, and are often used in addition to inhaled corticosteroids.

It has become very clear from clinical studies, however, that corticosteroids are the most effective medications for treating all but the mildest cases of asthma. Many comparative studies between corticosteroids and other medications have been performed. These studies consistently show that corticosteroids are superior to other medications. Corticosteroids improve air flow and ability to exercise, and reduce wheezing, shortness of breath, hospitalizations, and death more than any other medications tested to date.

Accordingly, corticosteroids have become the cornerstone of asthma therapy. There is universal agreement among experts and medical organizations that corticosteroids should be first-line treatment for asthma.

Do corticosteroids slow growth?

A number of studies have looked at rates of growth in children and teens with asthma. Determining the effects of corticosteroids can be difficult for a number of reasons. Severe asthma itself can affect growth, although in general, asthmatic children do not end up shorter than those without asthma. Because corticosteroids are so important in controlling asthma, it is ethically and practically difficult to study severely asthmatic people who do not receive inhaled corticosteroids. Therefore, nearly all studies have been performed in people with mild to moderate asthma symptoms.

The majority of studies have shown a small but significant reduction in growth velocity among children receiving inhaled steroids for asthma. This seems to be greatest in the first one to two years of use, and decreases as time goes on. Some studies have suggested that this effect may be stronger with some drugs than others. However, most experts feel that all inhaled corticosteroids have the potential to slow growth.

So, does this mean corticosteroids will make me shorter as an adult?

Interestingly, the answer appears to be no. Although the rate of growth may be somewhat slower with inhaled corticosteroids, multiple studies have concluded that there are little or no effects on final adult height.

Many studies have reported no difference in final height between asthmatic children who received inhaled corticosteroids and those who did not. Among those that did find a difference, the difference was very small: about one centimeter (less than half an inch).

♣ It's A Fact!!
Inhaled corticosteroids change your adult height by less than a half-inch.

Remember!!

- If you get short of breath more than twice a week, you probably need an inhaled corticosteroid.

- In people with asthma, the benefits of inhaled corticosteroids almost always outweigh their risks.

If corticosteroids slow growth velocity, why doesn't this mean shorter adult height?

This does seem like a contradiction. The studies don't tell us why treated children don't end up shorter, but there are some theories.

While children or teens initially grow more slowly on inhaled corticosteroids, it may be that they later "make up" for the lost growth near the start of treatment. It is also possible that teens on inhaled corticosteroids stop growing at a later age, so that slower growth is balanced by more time for growth.

What's the bottom line? Will inhaled steroids stunt my growth?

The evidence strongly indicates that inhaled corticosteroid use has little, if any, effects on their height as adults. Inhaled corticosteroid use will not stunt your growth.

Each person is different, and your treatment will need to be tailored to your individual needs. If your asthma requires high doses of inhaled corticosteroids, talk to your doctor about making regular growth measurements. Still, for the vast majority of asthmatics, the health benefits of inhaled corticosteroids far outweigh any known or theoretical risks.

Chapter 29

Dry Powder Inhalers

Asthma is a chronic inflammatory condition that causes the airways (bronchi) to produce excess mucus and close, making breathing difficult. Treatment has two main objectives: first, to control and reduce inflammation; and second, to reopen the airways. Drugs that achieve the first goal are called anti-inflammatory agents, and those that bring about the second are called bronchodilators. Many asthma sufferers inhale these medications. Following are answers to a few commonly asked questions about dry-powder inhalers.

What are the advantages of inhaling asthma medicines?

Anti-inflammatory treatment for asthma is long-term therapy. Often it is life long. Inhaling asthma medicine directly into airways and lungs has two advantages. First, the medicine goes directly to where it is needed and speeds relief of symptoms. And second, it limits the number of areas in the body exposed to the medicine and reduces the risk of side effects.

Are there different kinds of inhalers?

Yes, there are three basic types. The first type is the *nebulizer*. This is an electrical device that sends medicine directly into your mouth by tube or, in children, by clear mask. They require no hand-breath coordination. Simply put in the prescribed amount of medicine, take the tube in your mouth (or place the mask over the child's nose and mouth) and breathe normally until the medicine is gone.

The second type is the *metered-dose aerosol*. This sends a measured dose of medicine into your mouth using a small amount of pressurized gas. Sometimes a "spacer" is placed between the drug reservoir and your mouth to control the amount you inhale. Medicine is forced into the spacer, which you then squeeze as you inhale the medicine quickly. Aerosols fell out of favor a few years ago when the common propellant chlorofluorocarbon (CFC), a gas that depletes the atmosphere's ozone layer, was banned throughout the world.

The third type, the *dry-powder inhaler*, is a popular alternative to aerosols. It has the advantage of needing no propellant. But this is also a disadvantage. Because it has no propellant, it depends on the force of your inhalation to get medicine to your lungs. Children, people with severe asthma, and people suffering acute attacks may be unable to produce enough airflow to use dry-powder inhalers successfully.

What should I expect from my inhaler?

Inhaled anti-inflammatory drugs taken regularly should improve your breathing day and night, reducing the fear of having to struggle to breathe. They should reduce mucus production and, therefore, wheezing and coughing.

Inhaled bronchodilators will give you fast-acting, short-term relief from acute asthma symptoms caused by exercise or exposure to allergens if your asthma is mild to moderate.

What kinds of side effects might I experience?

In adults who use their inhalers only as prescribed, side effects are usually minor. Because the powder passes through your mouth on the way to your lungs, and because the particles are large, much of each dose (up to 90 percent) will deposit in your mouth or throat leaving a bad taste and perhaps irritating your tongue or throat. You can minimize this by rinsing your mouth after inhaling.

You may also swallow some of the medicine that remains after rinsing. This may cause minor stomach upset or "heartburn," which can do long-term damage. If it occurs, be sure to tell your doctor so it can be treated. Once absorbed in your stomach, swallowed asthma drugs are quickly eliminated from your body, so they don't have the widespread side effects of drugs taken as pills.

Can a child use a dry-powder inhaler?

Yes. Children five years old and up adjust easily to dry-powder inhalers, but they need careful instruction and watching to be certain they use them correctly. (Infants can use inhaled anti-inflammatory medicines by using nebulizers with masks.) Because of their low body weight, children's side effects are more dangerous for them than for adults. So despite the problems of teaching a child how to properly use an inhaler, this method of delivering medicine directly to the airways is preferred over pills for children.

♣ It's A Fact!!

People with severe asthma who take larger doses of anti-inflammatory medicines may have more serious side effects. A common one is a mouth or throat infection with yeast, called oral thrush, which appears as a white coating on the lining of the mouth and throat. This is easily treated.

Mature women who, because of severe asthma, take large doses of anti-inflammatory drugs may have a more serious side effect. These drugs can accelerate osteoporosis (a bone disease) after menopause. This can be checked by measuring bone density and, if osteoporosis is present, it can be treated with drugs that stimulate bone formation.

As with adults, children with asthma may need more than one inhaler. In order to run, swim, and play with others, a child with asthma may need one inhaler for constant anti-inflammatory treatment and another, containing different medicine, for bronchodilation when a child is involved in physical activity. This requires extra instruction from parents and the school nurse's awareness.

What are the side effects in children?

Even since anti-inflammatory therapy using corticosteroids was accepted as the front line treatment for asthma, including in children, researchers have debated its effect on growth. There is evidence that even low-dose, inhaled corticosteroids may temporarily delay a child's growth before puberty, slightly more in boys than in girls. After puberty, however, growth is regulated by sex hormones, and continued use of the steroid-based anti-inflammatory drugs has no additional impact. Ultimate height is not affected very much. Furthermore, the long-term benefits of these drugs greatly outweigh any minor effect on growth. Untreated asthma, in contrast, does cause reduction in final height.

There is newer evidence that anti-inflammatory medicines taken by dry-power inhaler may cause tooth erosion in children by changing the mouth's chemical environment. They also reduce the production of saliva, affecting the mouth's natural way of maintaining its chemical balance. To offset these side effects, some dentists recommend rinsing with a fluoride mouthwash and chewing sugarless gum to stimulate salivation after inhaling medicine. They recommend against brushing, because the action of brushing large-particle powder against young teeth may weaken already damaged enamel.

Who should use a dry-powder inhaler?

Almost anyone with asthma (more than 90 percent of all asthma patients) is usually able to inhale enough air to make the inhalers operate properly. The dry-powder inhalers are currently the most common inhalers. However, infants and toddlers, and anyone unable to manage the minimum hand-breath coordination needed for effective use, should not use this method. It also excludes anyone who, for any reason, is not responsible enough to use the inhaler as it is prescribed.

♣ It's A Fact!!

Dry-powder inhalers are a delivery system. Complications of asthma therapy come mostly from the medicines themselves, not from the delivery systems. Yet the way the drug is delivered may influence how well it works and the number of side effects. Nevertheless, except in emergency situations or unusual complications, inhaling asthma drugs has more benefits than side effects compared to any other form of medicine delivery method.

People with severe asthma, especially if confined to bed, may benefit more from the closed nebulizer system that provides constant airflow and uses smaller particles that get down to the airways more efficiently. But if you take asthma medicines that are not available in inhalable form you must, of course, continue to depend on pills or injections.

Are dry-powder inhalers beneficial?

Yes. They are convenient and easy to use. They dispense medicine directly to the place where it is needed, greatly reducing side effects as compared with medicines taken as pills or tablets. They also deliver medicine to the troubled site quickly, without need for absorption, digestion, and circulation. And they can deliver both long-lasting anti-inflammatory benefits or short-acting, quick-relief bronchodilation when needed. No other way of taking asthma drugs is so versatile.

Chapter 30

How To Use Asthma Medication Devices

Delivery Devices

Your doctor will prescribe the inhaler that is best suited for your needs. You may need to try a few different devices to see what is best for you. There are a variety of different medications and devices for delivering them. Reliever and controller medications may use the same type of device for delivery. Asthma medication is inhaled directly to the airways to treat the airway inflammation and bronchoconstriction so it is very important that you use them correctly to ensure maximum benefit of the medication. Proper inhaler techniques are covered later in this chapter.

The main types of inhalers are:

Metered Dose Inhalers (MDIs): This is likely the one you are most familiar with, also referred to as a 'puffer'. You inhale the medication as you push down on the canister in the sleeve which will deliver a preset dose. Examples of MDIs are: Ventolin, Flovent, Advair, Alvesco, Combivent, Airomir, and Qvar.

This medication should be used with a spacer for increased delivery to the airways. When your inhaler is used alone, medicine often ends up in your mouth, throat, stomach, and lungs. Medicine left in your mouth, throat, and stomach may cause unpleasant taste and side effects. When you use a drug delivery system (a spacer) with your inhaler, more medicine is delivered to your lungs.

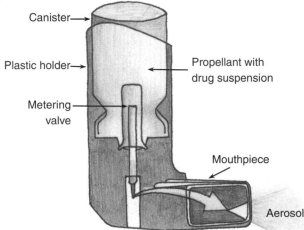

Figure 30.1. A metered dose inhaler looks like this.

A spacer helps get medicine to your lungs, where it works.

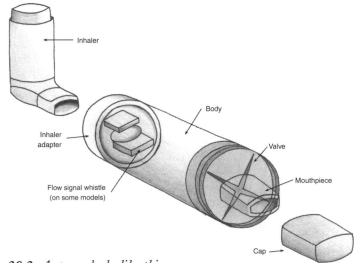

Figure 30.2. A spacer looks like this.

Turbuhalers: These devices deliver a dry powder medication as you breathe in. Loading this device is done by turning the dial at the bottom until you hear the 'click'. Examples of a Turbuhaler medication are Symbicort, Bricanyl, Pulmicort and Oxeze.

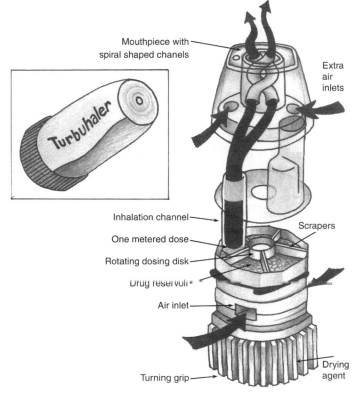

Mouthpiece with spiral shaped chanels

Extra air inlets

Inhalation channel

Scrapers

One metered dose

Rotating dosing disk

Drug reservoir

Air inlet

Turning grip

Drying agent

Figure 30.3. A Turbuhaler looks like this.

Diskus: This powder medication is inhaled from a device that resembles a 'hockey puck.' Loading the dose is done by opening the device, sliding the loading lever and inhaling from the mouthpiece. Examples of Diskus medications are Advair, Ventolin, Flovent and Serevent.

Remember to use your inhalers as directed by your physician. Review the use of your inhalers at your next visit with your doctor, asthma educator or pharmacist.

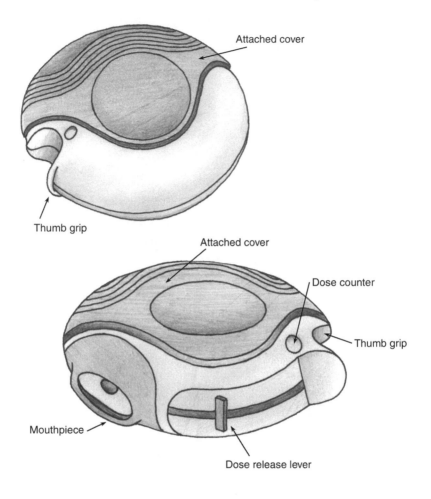

Figure 30.4. A Diskus looks like this.

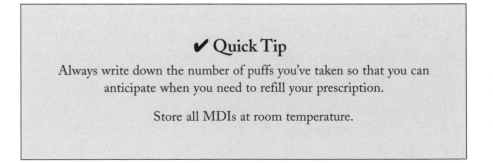

✔ Quick Tip

Always write down the number of puffs you've taken so that you can anticipate when you need to refill your prescription.

Store all MDIs at room temperature.

MDI Usage

You should follow the instructions packaged with your medication. The following is one way to use your inhaler.

To use your MDI without a spacer:

1. Shake the inhaler well before use (three or four shakes)

2. Remove the cap

3. Breathe out, away from your inhaler

4. Bring the inhaler to your mouth. Place it in your mouth between your teeth and close your mouth around it.

5. Start to breathe in slowly. Press the top of your inhaler once and keep breathing in slowly until you've taken a full breath

6. Remove the inhaler from your mouth, and hold your breath for about ten seconds, then breathe out.

If you need a second puff, wait 30 seconds, shake your inhaler again, and repeat steps 3–6.

Spacer With MDI Usage

Inhaled asthma medications are often delivered using a spacer or chamber. These devices have been shown to improve the delivery of drug directly to the airways. A spacer is a tube that you place your inhaler—a Metered Dose Inhaler (MDI) into and it holds the medication that is released (with activation of the MDI) until you can breathe it in. Many people do not use their inhaler correctly, or can not coordinate the MDI use, and the medication may collect in the mouth and/or throat.

There are a variety of spacing devices on the market, including sizes available for use with infants, young children, and adults. Speak with your health professional to determine which best meets your needs. Review the use of the spacer with your health care professional.

The spacer can be cleaned by soaking in a solution of mild detergent and lukewarm water for 15 minutes. Remove from solution and rinse with water.

Shake out the excess water and allow to air dry. Replace the device after 24 months of continuous use.

The Asthma Society recommends that anyone, of any age, using an MDI should consider using a spacer. Spacers are available for purchase from pharmacies.

To use your MDI with a spacer:

1.   Shake the inhaler well before use (three or four shakes)

2.   Remove the cap from your inhaler, and from your spacer, if it has one

---

♣ It's A Fact!!
The Transition To Ozone-Safe Propellants

What is happening with CFC-albuterol MDIs?

The U.S. Environmental Protection Agency (EPA) coordinates with the United States Food and Drug Administration (FDA) to determine which chlorofluorocarbon (CFC) metered-dose inhalers (MDIs) continue to be essential for public health as alternatives penetrate the market. In 2005, FDA removed the essential use designation for albuterol used in oral pressurized MDIs as of December 31, 2008. Therefore, after December 31, 2008, CFC-albuterol MDIs could not be sold, distributed or offered for sale or distribution in interstate commerce pursuant to Section 610 of the Clean Air Act (information on nonessential products ban). The term "interstate commerce" refers to the product's entire distribution chain up to, and including, the point of sale to the ultimate consumer.

Why are MDIs propelled by CFCs being phased out?

Chlorofluorocarbons (CFCs) deplete the stratospheric ozone layer. A thinner ozone layer allows more harmful ultraviolet (UV) radiation to reach the earth's surface. Overexposure to UV radiation can lead to serious health effects, such as skin cancer, cataracts, and immune suppression, as well serious ecological impacts.

The Montreal Protocol on Substances that Deplete the Ozone Layer (Montreal Protocol) is a landmark international agreement designed to protect

3. Put the inhaler into the spacer

4. Breathe out, away from the spacer

5. Bring the spacer to your mouth, put the mouthpiece between your teeth and close your lips around it

6. Press the top of your inhaler once

7. Breathe in slowly until you've taken a full breath. If you hear a whistle sound, you are breathing in too fast. Slowly breathe in.

8. Hold your breath for about ten seconds, then breathe out

---

the ozone layer. As a Party to the Montreal Protocol, the United States has committed to phasing out and eventually eliminating substances that deplete the ozone layer, including CFCs. It is estimated that actions to protect and restore the ozone layer will save an estimated 6.3 million U.S. lives that would have otherwise been lost to skin cancer.

The shift to CFC-free MDIs is part of a larger transition that has affected many consumer and industrial products and sectors over the last several decades. In 1996, the United States prohibited the production and import of CFCs except for certain essential uses. In fact, MDIs used for the treatment of asthma and chronic obstructive pulmonary disease were among the last uses to switch to ozone-safe alternatives.

Why do MDIs contain propellants?

MDIs use a chemical propellant to push medication out of the inhaler. Two common propellants are CFCs and HFAs (hydrofluoroalkanes). HFAs are ozone-safe propellants and are replacements for ozone-depleting CFCs in many sectors. Neither CFCs nor HFAs are medications; they serve only as the propellant that pushes the medication out of the inhaler. There are a variety of active medications that can be contained within MDIs, such as albuterol, flunisolide, cromolyn, and epinephrine.

Source: Excerpted from "Metered Dose Inhalers: The Transition to Ozone-Safe Propellants," U.S. Environmental Protection Agency (www.epa.gov), 2008.

Diskus® Usage

To use your DISKUS® do the following for one dose:

1. Open your DISKUS® and hold it in the palm of your hand, put the thumb of your other hand on the thumb grip and push the thumb grip until it clicks into place

2. Slide the lever away from you as far as it will go to get your medication ready

3. Breathe out away from the device

4. Place the mouthpiece gently in your mouth and close your lips around it

5. Breathe in deeply until you've taken a full breath

6. Remove the DISKUS® from your mouth

7. Hold your breath for about ten seconds, then breathe out slowly

Always check the number in the dose counter window to see how many doses are left.

Turbuhaler® Usage

To use your Turbuhaler®, do the following for one dose:

1. Unscrew the cap and take it off. Hold the inhaler upright.

2. Twist the colored grip of your Turbuhaler as far as it will go, then twist it all the way back. You've done it right when you hear a "click."

3. Breathe out away from the device

4. Put the mouthpiece between your teeth, and close your lips around it. Breathe in forcefully and deeply through your mouth

5. Remove the Turbuhaler from your mouth before breathing out

6. Always check the number in the dose counter window under the mouthpiece to see how many doses are left. For the Turbuhalers that do not have a dose counter window, check the window for a red mark, which means your medication is running out. When finished, replace the cap.

☞ Remember!!

Do not use a spacer with the DISKUS®, Turbuhaler® or any other dry powder inhaler.

Chapter 31

Alternative Therapies For Managing Asthma

What is alternative medicine?

Any unproven treatment for an illness or disease is considered an alternative medical approach by most American medical doctors. "Unproven" means there is not enough acceptable scientific evidence to show that the treatment works. The term *alternative medicine* refers to a wide variety of treatments considered outside "mainstream" or "usual" medical approaches in the United States today.

Why do people use alternative medicine?

Recent statistics show that nearly 40 percent of Americans try some form of alternative medicine. Medical and scientific experts do believe that some remedies may be worth a try, providing they are not harmful. In some cases, specific alternative medical treatment may improve or relieve symptoms of a specific illness or disease. Risks should not outweigh the potential benefits.

If you believe a particular alternative medical approach might help reduce your asthma or allergy symptoms, talk with your doctor about it, and how you could integrate that treatment into your overall asthma/allergy management plan.

Does health insurance cover alternative medical treatment?

Health plans vary in what alternative medicine expenses they will pay. Many plans provide coverage for some but not all alternative therapies. If your doctor writes you a prescription for a specific treatment such as acupuncture or massage, you may be more likely to get partial or full reimbursement of the expense. Always check with your insurance provider before assuming the coverage is available.

What are cautions or considerations for people who use alternative medicine?

Beware The Placebo Effect: If you really want an alternative medical treatment to work, you may think it is working, even if it really isn't. This "placebo effect" often occurs for people using alternative medicine. Symptoms of asthma or allergy also may improve on their own as an illness (like a cold or flu) runs its course. If you use prescribed medications for your allergy or asthma symptoms, it may take time for them to "kick in." So you may simply be feeling better because your medications started working—not because the alternative medicine is working.

♣ It's A Fact!!

Many people turn to alternative medicine to help alleviate their asthma or allergy symptoms. These treatment approaches may include, but are not limited to, one or more of the following:

- Acupuncture
- Ayurvedic medicine
- Biofeedback; mental imaging; stress reduction; relaxation techniques
- Chiropractic spinal manipulation
- Diet, exercise, yoga, lifestyle changes
- Herbal medicine, vitamin supplements
- Folk medicine from various cultures
- Laser therapy
- Massage
- Hypnosis
- Art or music therapy

Follow Directions: Never increase the amount or frequency of a dose or use a treatment or device in a different way than recommended. Do not use herbs in combinations. Do not take herbs if you are pregnant or breast feeding.

Beware Of Developing Allergy Symptoms: Allergies to specific plants and other substances (such as latex or nickel) can build up over time. Products you've used for years may suddenly cause mild to serious allergy symptoms, especially if you already are allergic to something. Check to see if new herbs, foods, or other products you plan to use are in the same "family" as your known allergens.

Use Quality Products And Services: Lack of quality standards is a serious problem for people who use various alternative medical treatments. Look for products that list the amount of the active ingredient(s). Make sure people giving you any kind of treatment are properly certified. Ask your pharmacist or health product store manager for recommendations. Research the product or service before you use it.

Consult With Your Physician Before Starting Any New Treatment: This point cannot be stressed enough. If you have symptoms of asthma or allergy, but you have not been diagnosed, consult a board-certified doctor for a proper diagnosis. Do not rely on health product store personnel to help treat undiagnosed symptoms. If you know you have asthma or allergies, again, talk with your doctor about the alternative medicine you want to use—before you try it.

Are there useful alternative therapies for people who have asthma or allergies?

Keep in mind: alternative therapy is medical treatment for which there is no conclusive, supporting scientific evidence. This does not necessarily mean the treatment is useless or ineffective. You simply must be careful in what you choose and how you use it.

☞ **Remember!!**

No one should use alternative medicine without first consulting a board-certified physician. Any alternative medical approach should be used in addition to your normal asthma or allergy management plan.

You should not substitute an alternative medical treatment for your regular medications or treatments. Be especially careful about use of alternative medicine on children. Approaches that are harmless for adults may not be harmless for children.

Acupuncture: A technique that involves inserting needles into key points of the body. Evidence suggests that acupuncture may signal the brain to release endorphins. These are hormones made by the body. When released, endorphins can help reduce pain and create a sense of well being. People with asthma or allergy may experience more relaxed or calmer breathing. Users should be aware of the risk of contaminated needles or punctured organs.

Biofeedback: A technique that helps people control involuntary physical responses. Results are mixed, with children and teenagers showing the greatest benefit.

Chiropractic Spinal Manipulation: A technique that emphasizes manipulation of the spine in order to help the body heal itself. There is no evidence that this treatment impairs the underlying disease or pulmonary function.

Hypnosis: An artificially induced dream state that leaves the person open to suggestion, hypnosis is a legitimate technique to help people manage various conditions. Hypnosis might give people with asthma or allergies more self-discipline to follow good health practices.

Laser Treatment: A technique that uses high intensity light to shrink swollen tissue or unblock sinuses. Laser therapy may provide temporary relief, but it may also cause scarring or other long-term physical problems.

Massage, Relaxation Techniques, Art/Music Therapy, Yoga: Stress and anxiety may cause your airways to constrict more if you have asthma or allergies. Various techniques can help you relax, reduce anxiety or control your breathing. The results may provide some benefit in helping you cope with asthma or allergy symptoms. However, evidence is not conclusive that these techniques improve lung function.

> ### ✔ Quick Tip
>
> Read between the label lines. The federal government requires labels to state how an herb or vitamin may affect the body, but labels are not required to carry health warnings. Labels also cannot claim any medical or health benefit. Products often are not properly labeled, especially those imported from other countries. Many people experience toxic—and sometimes deadly—effects from improperly using labeled herbs. Some products contain unnamed medicines such as steroids, anti-inflammatories or sedatives that act to reduce your symptoms. Other "hidden ingredients" in various products can be dangerous or even lethal. Use products tested for safety and effectiveness.

Part Four

Other Medical Conditions And Asthma

Chapter 32

Allergies And Asthma: What's The Connection?

Allergy Overview

Allergies are diseases of the immune system that cause an overreaction to substances called "allergens." Allergies are grouped by the kind of trigger, time of year, or where symptoms appear on the body: indoor and outdoor allergies (also called "hay fever," "seasonal," "perennial" or "nasal" allergies), food and drug allergies, latex allergies, insect allergies, skin allergies, and eye allergies. People who have allergies can live healthy and active lives.

What are allergies?

Allergies reflect an overreaction of the immune system to substances that usually cause no reaction in most individuals. These substances can trigger sneezing, wheezing, coughing, and itching. Allergies are not only bothersome, but many have been linked to a variety of common and serious chronic respiratory illnesses (such as sinusitis and asthma). Additionally, allergic reactions can be severe and even fatal. However, with proper management and patient education, allergic diseases can be controlled, and people with allergies can lead normal and productive lives.

About This Chapter: This chapter includes text from "Allergy Overview" and "Living With Allergic Asthma," © 2005 Asthma and Allergy Foundation of America (www.aafa.org). All rights reserved. Reprinted with permission.

Common Allergic Diseases

Allergic Rhinitis (hay fever or "indoor/outdoor," "seasonal," "perennial" or "nasal" allergies): Characterized by nasal stuffiness, sneezing, nasal itching, clear nasal discharge, and itching of the roof of the mouth and/or ears.

Allergic Asthma (asthma symptoms triggered by an allergic reaction): Characterized by airway obstruction that is at least partially reversible with medication and is always associated with allergy. Symptoms include coughing, wheezing, shortness of breath or rapid breathing, chest tightness, and occasional fatigue and slight chest pain.

Food Allergy: Most prevalent in very young children and frequently outgrown, food allergies are characterized by a broad range of allergic reactions. Symptoms may include itching or swelling of lips or tongue; tightness of the throat with hoarseness; nausea and vomiting; diarrhea; occasional chest tightness and wheezing; itching of the eyes; decreased blood pressure, or loss of consciousness and anaphylaxis.

Drug Allergy: Drug allergy is characterized by a variety of allergic responses affecting any tissue or organ. Drug allergies can cause anaphylaxis; even those patients who do not have life-threatening symptoms initially may progress to a life-threatening reaction.

Anaphylaxis (extreme response to a food or drug allergy): Characterized by life-threatening symptoms. This is a medical emergency and the most severe form of allergic reaction. Symptoms include a sense of impending doom; generalized warmth or flush; tingling of palms, soles of feet or lips; lightheadedness; bloating and chest tightness. These can progress into seizures, cardiac arrhythmia, shock, and respiratory distress. Possible causes can be medications, vaccines, food, latex, and insect stings and bites.

Latex Allergy: An allergic response to the proteins in natural, latex rubber characterized by a range of allergic reactions. Persons at risk include healthcare workers, patients having multiple surgeries, and rubber-industry workers. Symptoms include hand dermatitis, eczema, and urticaria; sneezing and other respiratory distress; and lower respiratory problems including coughing, wheezing, and shortness of breath.

Insect Sting/Bite Allergy: Characterized by a variety of allergic reactions; stings cannot always be avoided and can happen to anyone. Symptoms include pain, itching and swelling at the sting site or over a larger area and can cause anaphylaxis. Insects that sting include bees, hornets, wasps, yellow jackets, and fire and harvest ants.

Urticaria (hives, skin allergy): A reaction of the skin, or a skin condition commonly known as *hives*. Characterized by the development of itchy, raised white bumps on the skin surrounded by an area of red inflammation. Acute urticaria is often caused by an allergy to foods or medication.

Atopic Dermatitis (eczema, skin allergy): A chronic or recurrent inflammatory skin disease characterized by lesions, scaling, and flaking; it is sometimes called *eczema*. In children, it may be aggravated by an allergy or irritant.

Contact Dermatitis (skin allergy): Characterized by skin inflammation; this is the most common occupational disease representing up to 40 percent of all occupational illnesses. Contact dermatitis is one of the most common skin diseases in adults. It results from the direct contact with an outside substance with the skin. There are currently about 3,000 known contact allergens.

Allergic Conjunctivitis (eye allergy): Characterized by inflammation of the eyes; it is the most common form of allergic eye disease. Symptoms can include itchy and watery eyes and lid distress. Allergic conjunctivitis is also commonly associated with the presence of other allergic diseases such as atopic dermatitis, allergic rhinitis, and asthma.

What causes allergies?

The substances that cause allergic disease in people are known as *allergens*. "Antigens," or protein particles like pollen, food, or dander enter our bodies through a variety of ways. If the antigen causes an allergic reaction, that particle is considered an "allergen"—an antigen that triggers an allergic reaction. These allergens can get into our body in several ways:

- Inhaled into the nose and the lungs. Examples are airborne pollens of certain trees, grasses and weeds; house dust that include dust mite particles, mold spores, cat and dog dander, and latex dust.

- Ingested by mouth. Frequent culprits include shrimp, peanuts, and other nuts.

- Injected. Such as medications delivered by needle like penicillin or other injectable drugs, and venom from insect stings and bites.

- Absorbed through the skin. Plants such as poison ivy, sumac and oak, and latex are examples.

What makes some pollen cause allergies, and not others?

Plant pollens that are carried by the wind cause most allergies of the nose, eyes, and lungs. These plants (including certain weeds, trees, and grasses) are natural pollutants produced at various times of the year when their small, inconspicuous flowers discharge literally billions of pollen particles.

♣ It's A Fact!!

Allergic Asthma Triggers

With allergic asthma, certain types of allergens are known to produce, or trigger, asthma symptoms and attacks. Triggers cause symptoms in allergic asthma often associated with a substance made by the body called immunoglobulin E (IgE). If you have allergic asthma, your body makes more IgE when you breathe an allergen. This can cause a series of chemical reactions known as the allergic-inflammatory process in allergic asthma, resulting in the constriction (tightening) and inflammation (swelling) of the airways in your lungs.

Common Triggers Of Allergic Asthma

The following allergens are well-known triggers of coughing, wheezing, tightening of the chest, and other symptoms of allergic asthma. For tips on reducing your exposure to allergens, see "Living with Allergic Asthma" later in this chapter.

Cockroaches: Cockroach feces and saliva are both allergens and can trigger asthma symptoms in some people with allergic asthma. Because cockroaches are often prevalent in many inner-city areas, their allergens play a significant role in contributing to the number of people with asthma.

Dust Mites: Dust mites are spider-like creatures too small to see with the naked eye. Every home has dust mites. They feed on skin flakes and are found

Because the particles can be carried significant distances, it is important for you not only to understand local environmental conditions, but also conditions over the broader area of the state or region in which you live. Unlike the wind-pollinated plants, conspicuous wild flowers or flowers used in most residential gardens are pollinated by bees, wasps, and other insects and therefore are not widely capable of producing allergic disease.

What is the role of heredity in allergy?

Like baldness, height, and eye color, the capacity to become allergic is an inherited characteristic. Yet, although you may be born with the genetic capability to become allergic, you are not automatically allergic to specific allergens. Several factors must be present for allergic sensitivity to be developed:

in mattresses, pillows, carpets, upholstered furniture, bedcovers, clothes, stuffed toys, fabric, etc. Both the body parts and feces of dust mites can trigger asthma in individuals with an allergic reaction to dust mites.

Mold: Molds can grow on virtually anything when moisture is present. Outdoors, many molds live in soil, or on leaves, wood, and other plant debris. Indoors, they can grow on wood, paper, carpet, and food. Molds produce tiny spores, which are like seeds, to reproduce. These spores become airborne easily. Any time moisture accumulates indoors (through a damp basement, leaky faucet, shower stall, etc.), mold growth will often occur, particularly if the excess moisture goes unnoticed or unaddressed. Asthma episodes can be triggered in individuals with an allergic reaction to mold.

Pet Dander: Asthma can be triggered by pet urine, feces, saliva, hair, or dander (skin flakes). But you don't have to have pets in your house or visit places where animals are kept in order to be exposed to their allergens. Interestingly enough, animal allergens are often detected in places where no animals are housed. The allergens may have been carried unwittingly into a place by people that own or have been around animals.

- The specific genes acquired from parents

- The exposure to one or more allergens to which you have a genetically programmed response

- The degree and length of exposure

A baby born with the tendency to become allergic to cow's milk, for example, may show allergic symptoms several months after birth. A genetic capability to become allergic to cat dander may take three to four years of cat exposure before the person shows symptoms. These people may also become allergic to other environmental substances with age.

On the other hand, poison ivy allergy (contact dermatitis) is an example of an allergy in which hereditary background does not play a part. The person with poison ivy allergy first has to be exposed to the oil from the plant. This usually occurs during youth, when a rash does not always appear. However, the first exposure may sensitize or cause the person to become allergic and, when subsequent exposure takes place, a contact dermatitis rash appears and can be quite severe. Many plants are capable of producing this type of rash. Substances other than plants, such as dyes, metals, and chemicals in deodorants and cosmetics, can also cause a similar dermatitis.

Diagnosis

If you break out in hives when a bee stings you, or you sneeze every time you pet a cat, you know what some of your allergens are. But if the pattern is not so obvious, try keeping a record of when, where, and under what circumstances your reactions occur. This can be as easy as jotting down notes on a calendar. If the pattern still isn't clear, make an appointment with your doctor for help.

Doctors diagnose allergies in three steps:

1. Personal and medical history. Your doctor will ask you questions to get a complete understanding of your symptoms and their possible causes. Bring your notes to help jog your memory. Be ready to answer questions about your family history, the kinds of medicines you take, and your lifestyle at home, school, and work.

2. Physical examination. If your doctor suspects an allergy, he or she will pay special attention to your ears, eyes, nose, throat, chest, and skin during the physical examination. This exam may include a pulmonary function test to detect how well you exhale air from your lungs. You may also need an x-ray of your lungs or sinuses.

3. Tests to determine your allergens. Your doctor may do a skin test, patch test, or blood test.

Skin Test: For most people, skin tests are the most accurate and least expensive way to confirm suspected allergens. There are two types of allergen skin tests. In prick/scratch testing, a small drop of the possible allergen is placed on the skin, followed by lightly pricking or scratching with a needle through the drop. In intradermal (under the skin) testing, a very small amount of allergen is injected into the outer layer of skin.

With either test, if you are allergic to the substance, you will develop redness, swelling, and itching at the test site within 20 minutes. You may also see a "wheal" or raised, round area that looks like a hive. Usually, the larger the wheal, the more sensitive you are to the allergen.

Patch Test: This test determines if you have contact dermatitis. Your doctor will place a small amount of a possible allergen on your skin, cover it with a bandage, and check your reaction after 48 hours. If you are allergic to the substance, you should develop a rash.

✔ Quick Tip
Avoiding Your Allergens

The best way to prevent allergy symptoms and minimize your need for allergy medicine is to avoid your allergens as much as possible and to eliminate the source of allergens from your home and other environments. For important tips, talk to your doctor.

Source: From "Allergy Overview," © 2005 Asthma and Allergy Foundation of America.

Blood Tests: Allergen blood tests (also called radioallergosorbent tests [RAST], enzyme-linked immunosorbent assays [ELISA], fluorescent allergosorbent tests [FAST], multiple radioallergosorbent tests [MAST], or radioimmunosorbent tests [RIST]) are sometimes used when people have a skin condition or are taking medicines which interfere with skin testing. Your doctor will take a blood sample and send it to a laboratory. The lab adds the allergen to your blood sample, and then measures the amount of antibodies your blood produces to attack the allergens.

Treatment

Good allergy treatment is based on the results of your allergy tests, your medical history, and the severity of your symptoms. It can include three different treatment strategies: avoidance of allergens, medication options, and/or immunotherapy (allergy shots).

Medication

Some people don't take allergy medicines because they don't take their symptoms seriously ("Oh, it's only my allergies.") The result may be painful complications such as sinus or ear infections. Don't take the risk. There are so many safe prescription and non-prescription medicines to relieve allergy symptoms. Following is a brief list of medications taken for allergies. They are available in non-prescription and prescription form.

- *Antihistamines* and *decongestants* are the most common medicines used for allergies. Antihistamines help relieve rashes and hives, as well as sneezing, itching, and runny nose. Prescription antihistamines are similar to their non-prescription counterparts, but many of them do not cause drowsiness. Decongestant pills, sprays, and nose drops reduce stuffiness by shrinking swollen membranes in the nose.

  It is important to remember that using a non-prescription nasal decongestant spray more than three days in a row may cause the swelling and stuffiness in your nose to become worse, even after you stop using the medicine. This is called a "rebound" reaction. Some non-prescription "cold" medicines combine an antihistamine, a pain reliever like aspirin or acetaminophen, and a decongestant. Aspirin can cause asthma attacks in some people. Don't take a chance: if you have asthma, talk with your doctor before taking any non-prescription allergy medicine.

- *Eye drops* may provide temporary relief from burning or bloodshot eyes. However, only prescription allergy eye drops contain antihistamines that can reduce itching, tearing, and swelling.

- *Corticosteroid creams* or ointments relieve itchiness and halt the spread of rashes. Corticosteroids are not the same as anabolic steroids that are used illegally by some athletes to build muscles. If your rash does not go away after using a non-prescription corticosteroid for (a week?), see your doctor.

- *Corticosteroid nasal sprays* help reduce the inflammation that causes nasal congestion without the chance of the "rebound" effect found in non-prescription nose sprays.

- *Cromolyn sodium* prevents the inflammation which causes nasal congestion. Because it has few, if any, side effects, cromolyn can be safely used over long periods of time.

- *Oral corticosteroids* may be prescribed to reduce swelling and stop severe allergic reactions. Because these medications can cause serious side effects, you should expect your doctor to carefully monitor you.

- *Epinephrine* comes in pre-measured, self-injectable containers, and is the only medication which can help during a life-threatening anaphylactic attack. To be effective, epinephrine must be given within minutes of the first sign of serious allergic reaction.

Note: New prescription and non-prescription drugs are approved periodically. If the prescription you are taking is not on this list, ask your doctor which category (above) it falls into, so that you can refer to this information.

Living With Allergic Asthma

Make life with allergic asthma a little easier by avoiding the things you're allergic to. Sound like common sense? Sure it does. Unfortunately, trying to put this advice into practice in your everyday life is not always practical. For example, in order to completely avoid ragweed pollen, you couldn't go outdoors from August to November. There are, however, a few steps you can take that are more realistic and can be very helpful.

To help lessen the allergic reactions that cause your asthma symptoms, familiarize yourself with the following strategies for avoiding allergens from cockroaches, dust mites, mold spores, and pet dander.

Cockroaches

- Limit where you eat to avoid spreading food and crumbs around the house and always keep food out of bedrooms.
- Never leave food out—keep all food and garbage in closed containers.
- Wash the kitchen floor and countertops at least once a week.
- Repair leaky faucets and drain pipes to eliminate water sources that attract these pests.
- Close up all openings around the house that might allow cockroaches to enter.
- Reduce the number of cockroaches by using environmentally safe pesticides and bait stations.

Dust Mites

- Encase your mattress and pillows in dust-proof or allergen impermeable covers (available from mail-order specialty supply companies, as well as some bedding and department stores).
- Wash all bedding and blankets once a week in hot water (at least 130–140° F) to kill dust mites.

- Replace wool or feathered bedding with synthetic materials, and make sure all stuffed animals are washable.

- If possible, replace wall-to-wall carpets in bedrooms with bare floors (linoleum, tile, or wood).

- Use a damp mop or rag to remove dust from surfaces. Never use a dry cloth, which just stirs up mite allergens.

- Use a dehumidifier or air conditioner to maintain relative humidity at 50 percent or below.

- Use a vacuum cleaner with either a double-layered microfilter bag or a high-efficiency particulate air (HEPA) filter to trap allergens that pass through a vacuum's exhaust.

Mold Spores

- Use a dehumidifier or air conditioner to maintain relative humidity below 50 percent and keep temperatures cool.

- Vent clothes dryers and bathrooms to the outside so that moisture does not accumulate in your home.

- Check faucets, pipes, and ductwork for leaks.

- After you turn on air conditioners in your home or car, leave the room or drive with the windows open for several minutes to allow mold spores to disperse.

- Remove decaying debris from the yard, roof, and gutters.

- Avoid raking leaves, mowing lawns, and working with peat, mulch, hay, or dead wood. If you must do yard work, wear a mask and avoid working on hot, humid days.

Pet Dander

- If possible, remove all pets from your home.

- If it is not possible to remove pets, keep them confined to areas without carpets or upholstered furniture and out of bedrooms.

- When near any rodents (mice, hamsters, guinea pigs, squirrels, etc.), wear a dust mask and gloves.

- Wash your hands and clean your clothes after playing with your pet—this will remove pet allergens.

- When possible, ask someone else to clean soiled litter cages.

- Dust regularly with a damp cloth.

Chapter 33

Chronic Obstructive Pulmonary Disease (COPD)

What Is COPD?

Chronic obstructive pulmonary disease, or COPD, is a term used to describe two diseases that affect the lungs—chronic bronchitis and emphysema. COPD causes progressive damage to the lungs.

COPD Facts

Over 16 million Americans have been diagnosed with COPD and another 16 million have COPD but don't know it (have not been diagnosed). This means that over 32 million Americans suffer from COPD.

COPD Is A Serious Health Problem

- COPD is the fourth leading cause of death in the U.S.

- In a recent survey, seven out of 10 smokers could not identify COPD as a top-five killer.

- In 2002, about 125,000 people died of COPD.

About This Chapter: Text in this chapter is from "Lung Diseases: COPD," © 2005 American Association for Respiratory Care (http://www.yourlunghealth.org). Reprinted with permission.

- While other chronic health diseases such as heart disease and diabetes have decreased in the past 20 years, COPD rates have steadily increased.

- In a recent survey 66 percent of Americans did not know that COPD kills more women than men.

- COPD will continue to be a major health problem in the future. By 2020, COPD will become the third leading cause of death in the United States.

COPD Does Not Sexually Discriminate

- Women who smoke are more susceptible to developing COPD than are men.

- Women may develop COPD at an earlier age and with less duration or intensity of smoking.

- U.S. women had more COPD hospitalizations (404,000) than men (322,000) and also had more emergency department visits (898,000) than men (551,000) in 2000.

- 66 percent of Americans did not know that COPD kills more women than men.

- More women than men die of COPD.

Table 33.1. 32 Million Have COPD in the U.S.

Emphysema	Chronic Bronchitis	Undiagnosed	Total
2,000,000	14,000,000	16,000,000	32,000,000

Table 33.2. Asthma vs. COPD Deaths

Asthma: 4,261   COPD: 125,000

Decrease Your Risk For COPD

- Do not smoke

- Quit smoking

- Stay away from second-hand smoke

- Wear a mask or respirator when working around dust, chemicals, paints and solvents (varnish, paint thinners, adhesives, inks, refrigerant/coolants, etc.)

- Limit outdoor activity when ozone levels are high; check with the Environmental Protection Agency (EPA) for daily ozone levels across the U.S.

♣ It's A Fact!!
Causes Of COPD

- Cigarette smoking is the leading cause of COPD

- Smoking a pipe, cigar, marijuana, hashish and other types of smoking materials

- Breathing in second-hand smoke

- Working around certain kinds of chemicals and breathing in the fumes for many years

- Working in a dusty area for many years

- Having heavy exposure to air pollution

- Having a history of frequent childhood lung infections

- Having the genetic disorder alpha 1 antitrypsin deficiency

Get to Know Your Healthy Lungs

Knowledge Is Power: Take the time to learn about healthy lungs. It will help you to understand how COPD damages the lungs and how this lung damage affects the daily life of someone with COPD. Having a clear picture of what effect COPD has on the lungs will help you to maintain and improve your lungs health.

People with normal healthy lungs breathe 12–18 times a minute, that's 20,000 time a day.

Oxygen is delivered to the lungs with each breath. Oxygen is your body's fuel to maintain growth and repair every cell in your body. You need healthy lungs to keep your body working like it should.

What Does The Outside Of The Lungs Look Like?

You have a right and a left lung. Your heart sits in between the two lungs. The right lung is the larger lung and it has three distinct parts called lobes. There is an upper, middle, and lower lobe.

The left lung is smaller, as it has to make room for the heart. The left lung has only two lobes—the upper and lower lobe.

The Muscles Of Breathing

The diaphragm is the large curved muscle located below your lungs. It is the main muscle used in breathing. When the diaphragm drops down (contracts) and the rib cage expands, the air flows into the lungs. When the lungs are full of air, the diaphragm relaxes (goes back to its original position) and air is pushed out of your lungs.

There are other muscles in your neck and in between your ribs that also can help with breathing.

Smooth Muscle: When you have COPD, the smooth muscles become stretched out; making it harder to breathe out all of your air. You may "trap" air in your lungs meaning that not all the air is exhaled from the lungs.

Asthma is a little different. In asthma, the muscles of the airway tighten up (spasm) and your airways become narrow—and again it is hard to get the air out of the lungs. With asthma the airway muscles are not stretched out.

Working together, all the muscles cause pressure changes inside of the lung that in turn helps move the air in and out of your lungs. Most of the time, people with healthy lungs do not have to think about breathing. Those with lung diseases have to work to breathe.

Moving The Air In And Out Of The Lungs

Think of your lungs and airways as branches on a tree. Each breath you take enters the mouth or nose and travels down the windpipe (trachea) and into the two large airways (bronchi) that lead to the right or left lung.

Once the air enters the lungs, it goes through 22 smaller and smaller tubes until it reaches the tiniest tubes called the bronchioles. You have over 100,000 of them.

Finally the airflow travels from the bronchioles down to the 1,000,000 tiny air sacs (alveoli). These little air sacs look like clusters of grapes.

It is here in the alveoli where the oxygen (fuel) is delivered to the bloodstream and the carbon dioxide (waste) is removed. This process happens every time you take a breath and let it out.

What Keeps The Lungs Inflated

The lungs are in a cavity that is protected by the ribs. The glue, so to speak, that keeps the lungs inflated is called the "pleura." The pleura are two thin linings or membranes that protect and cushion the lungs.

One lining covers the lungs. It is called the *visceral pleura*—the other lining covers the chest wall, it is called the *parietal pleura*.

Between these two linings there is a small amount of fluid (pleural fluid) that lubricates the surface of the linings, so the two surfaces glide smoothly over each other.

It might be helpful to think of the linings as two pieces of glass placed on top of each other, one representing the lung pleural and the other piece being the chest wall pleural. If you set these pieces of glass one on top of the other they can easily be separated. But if you lightly coat the inside glass with water (pleural fluid), the pieces slide easily over each other and it becomes very difficult to separate the pieces of glass.

Take A Look Inside The Lungs

The lung resembles a sponge with tiny holes. It is made up of 90 percent blood and 10 percent tissue.

Your lungs work best when they are clean. Keeping the lungs clean is very important in preventing infections and delivering oxygen to the body.

Normal, healthy lungs produce thin, clear mucus (a sticky fluid) to protect the lungs. When something irritates the lungs (dirt, fumes, or smoke) the lungs make more mucus to protect the delicate lung tissue.

Tiny hair-like structures, called *cilia*, beat fast enough to move the mucus up the airways. As the mucus moves up the airways, irritants stick to the mucus and it is removed with a cough or is swallowed.

Smoking damages the cilia. The useless cilia cannot move the mucus up the airways and as a result, mucus builds up in the lungs and becomes quite thick. This type of situation leaves the lungs vulnerable to infections.

Irritants remain in the lungs when the cilia are damaged. The airways become swollen and narrow when irritants stay in the lungs for an extended period of time.

Over time, irritants that are not removed can destroy the lung's elastic ability, and the lungs become floppy, making breathing harder. The loss of elasticity decreases the lungs ability to exhale and air remains trapped inside of the lungs.

COPD In A Nut Shell

Bronchitis And Acute Bronchitis: Bronchitis is an inflammation (thickening and/or swelling) of the lining of the bronchi and increased mucus production. Inflammation can be caused by smoke, infections, chemicals, pollution, and/or acids from your stomach (gastroesophageal reflux disease, GERD).

Many people have had a brief attack of bronchitis, often after you have had a cold. The attack usually lasts for about a week, but the cough may last up to three weeks. During a bout with bronchitis, you may experience cough with large amounts of mucus production, and sometimes a fever.

This brief type of bronchitis is called Acute Bronchitis—each attack does not last long and does not come back again and again. Lung function returns to normal after the bronchitis infection has ended.

♣ **It's A Fact!!**

Other diseases with similar symptoms of chronic bronchitis:

- Infection
- Tuberculosis
- Lung cancer
- Congestive heart failure

Acute bronchitis is not COPD.

Chronic Bronchitis: Chronic bronchitis is an ongoing illness that can cause serious long-lasting lung problems. The signs and symptoms of chronic bronchitis are:

- a cough with mucus production that lasts at least for three months;

- the productive cough is present for two years in a row.

Of course other diseases must be excluded before chronic bronchitis can be diagnosed.

Chronic bronchitis is a condition when repeated lung inflammation damages the lungs. Chronic inflammation in the lungs causes scarring of the airways and excessive production of mucus that results in a chronic cough. Some call it a "smoker's" cough.

As the lining of the airways becomes thickened and narrow or obstructed (due to the scarring) less air is moved in and out of the lungs. Air becomes trapped in the lungs and this limits the amount of air that you are able to breathe in with each breath.

If the inflammation continues and the cough becomes more regular (a daily event rather than just periods of coughing) this can progress to the point where shortness of breath is present. Chronic bronchitis can exist alone, before, or during emphysema.

COPD has no cure, yet there are treatments, along with the removal of irritants, that will decrease the effects of COPD.

Emphysema: Emphysema develops when many of the small air sacs or alveoli in the lungs get stretched out and lose their ability to empty out all of the air. Air becomes trapped in the alveoli and the alveoli become stretched out and over-inflated.

This damage can cause the alveoli to come apart (rupture), and form one large air space instead of many small ones. The destruction of healthy air sacs makes it difficult for the lung to work properly.

There are less alveoli to deliver oxygen to the bloodstream. The damage is progressive and, as lung tissue does not repair itself, the damage is permanent. The whole body suffers when the lung cannot deliver the essential oxygen and remove the carbon dioxide waste.

The increased pressure of the trapped air, over time, will shorten and flatten the diaphragm. This change in the shape of the diaphragm makes it much harder for the diaphragm to play its part in moving air in and out of the lungs. The diaphragm muscle becomes weak and fatigued.

An additional result of the trapped air is that the chest cavity becomes larger (barrel chest) and the muscles in between the ribs become stretched out.

The change in the muscles of breathing significantly increase the work of breathing. Normally, the muscles of breathing require a low level of oxygen at rest (one to three percent) but when you have COPD, the needed oxygen increases to as high as 25 percent.

Symptoms Of COPD

The main cause of COPD is smoking tobacco. Years of smoking can cause damage to the airways of the lungs. Many current and former smokers will probably not notice or will simply not accept symptoms for several years.

Symptoms of COPD are:

- cough;
- extreme mucus production;
- shortness of breath, especially with exercise;
- wheezing (a whistling or squeaky sound when you breathe);
- chest tightness.

These symptoms are due to permanent airway obstruction caused by airway inflammation. The reduced airflow hurts the lung's ability to deliver oxygen to the body and to remove carbon dioxide waste.

COPD sufferers become short of breath because of the increased effort needed to breathe. When you have COPD it becomes 'work' to move the air in and out of your lungs.

The feeling of shortness of breath causes changes in the way you live your life. You may need to adapt your activities to help decrease the shortness of breath.

Physical activities may take longer to complete. The person with COPD may take frequent rest periods in order to be able to complete an activity, such as vacuuming, mowing a yard, or cooking a meal.

Diagnosing COPD

Early Detection Of COPD: It is hard to diagnosis COPD in the early stages. Many times COPD symptoms are ignored or thought to be "just being out of shape" or part of "getting older."

Usually, those with COPD will begin to notice symptoms of shortness of breath when they reach their mid-40s. However, early signs of COPD (chronic cough and increased mucus production) may be present but are not bad enough to cause concern.

However, the earlier you know you have COPD, the earlier you and your doctor can take steps to improve your lung health and to prevent further damage to the airway. Some measures such as smoking cessation and avoiding respiratory irritants can help you stop the damage to your lungs.

Spirometry: Spirometry is used to diagnose and monitor the progress of COPD. According to the National Lung Health Education Program, all persons aged 45 or older who currently smoke or have quit smoking should have a spirometry test.

The test is done in the doctor's office and takes only a few minutes to complete. You will be asked to take a deep breath in and then blow out all the air in your lungs as hard and fast as you can for at least six seconds.

After the test is completed, the doctor will look at two important numbers:

- FEV1: The amount of air that is blown out in the first second of exhalation
- FEV1/FEV6: A ratio of the time it takes you to blow out one second to the amount of air that you can blow out in six seconds. This number

(written as a percent) gives the doctor important information needed to make the diagnosis of COPD.

Do I Need To Be Tested For COPD?

- Do you (now) or have you ever smoked?

- Are you short of breath more often than other people?

- Do you have a cough that does not go away? For example: daily coughing or the 'morning' cough?

- If you cough, do you cough up mucus?

- Do people around you smoke?

- Do you work around chemicals and dust?

- Does bronchitis or emphysema run in your family?

- Do you wheeze? (a whistling or squeaky sound when you breathe)

If you have answered, "yes" to any one of these questions, ask your doctor about having a simple breathing test to check for COPD.

COPD and asthma have some of the same symptoms, such as coughing and wheezing. But there some important differences between the two such as:

- COPD most often develops in smokers and former smokers who are in their mid-40s;

- the age of onset of COPD for those who have alpha 1 emphysema is usually between 30 to 40 years of age;

- asthma occurs at all ages and it is more common in children than adults;

- a flare-up of COPD is often caused by respiratory tract infections— often seen symptoms are: decreased energy level making your usual activities harder to complete, increased mucus production, change in color of mucus, increased coughing;

- COPD patients rarely have a day without symptoms. Airflow obstruction in COPD is only partially reversible with smoking cessation and bronchodilator use. Medications do help, but the airways are never quite normal.

- with medication, asthma patients have near-normal lung function and are symptom-free between flare-ups.

COPD Flare-Ups

What Happens With A Flare-Up?

Lung infections and airway irritations cause an increase in the symptoms of COPD:

- Increased coughing and mucus production
- Change in mucus color and shortness of breath, possibly with wheezing

Flare-ups (the medical term is *exacerbations*) are the result of lung infections or irritation. The increased amount of mucus decreases the lungs' ability to clear the mucus, and airflow becomes more obstructed (airflow slows down). As the FEV1 falls, emergency room visits and hospitalization are more likely to be used.

Dangers Of Flare-Ups

A flare-up can be life threatening and early action is needed to stop the flare-up before it becomes deadly. It is important to avoid situations that increase your chances of getting an infection such as crowded malls and places where people are coughing and sneezing.

You need to be aware of changes in your "normal" condition and immediately report any signs of a flare-up to your doctor. Remember some flare-ups come on quickly and others slowly develop so don't delay making the call to your doctor. Quick reaction to flare-ups could greatly reduce the risk of deadly complications.

Events And Symptoms That Are Often Seen With Flare-Ups

- Increased shortness of breath
- Not feeling well. Your usual daily activities may be more tiring and require more physical effort.
- Increased amount of your 'normal' mucus production. It may also be thicker and greenish in color.

- Recent viral or bacterial infection

- Wheezing

- Exposure to high pollution levels

- Exposure to irritants: chemicals, smoke, dust, etc.

- Fever

Treatment Of Flare-Ups

Although about 30 percent of flare-ups are viral infections, antibiotics are used when signs and symptoms of a flare-up are present. Changes in your routine bronchodilator therapy may be necessary until the flare-up is under control. Finally, corticoid steroid (orally or inhaled) may be used to control the inflammation in the airways.

Treatment Of COPD

Goals Of Treatment

COPD is not a curable disease, but it is treatable. Instead of trying to cure COPD the focus of treatment is to:

- slow down the damage to the lung;

- relieve symptoms, such as shortness of breath and cough;

- build up overall body fitness;

- decrease flare-ups;

- improve quality of life.

Stop Smoking: The most important step in treating COPD is to *stop smoking*. Smoking causes a progressive loss of lung function.

When you quit, you stop the damage to the lung and your lung function may improve with time. Everyone can benefit from not smoking, no matter how old you are.

Chapter 34

Colds And Influenza

Flu (Influenza)

The flu is a contagious respiratory illness caused by influenza viruses. It can cause mild to severe illness, and can lead to death in severe cases. For people with asthma, guarding against the flu is important every year because your lung function can be very compromised if you catch the flu, making your asthma symptoms even worse.

Most healthy people recover from the flu without complications, some people, such as older people, young children, and people with certain health conditions like asthma, are at high risk for serious complications from the flu. Some of the complications caused by the flu include bacterial pneumonia, dehydration, and worsening of existing chronic conditions, such as congestive heart failure, asthma, or diabetes. Children and adults could also develop sinus problems or ear infections.

People at high risk for complications include people 65 years or older, people with chronic medical conditions, pregnant women, and young children. If you are at high risk from complications of the flu, you should consult your health-care provider to learn how to prevent the flu. If you develop flu-like symptoms, seek professional medical help.

About This Chapter: This chapter includes text from "Flu (Influenza)," © 2009 Asthma and Allergy Foundation of America, and "Flu/Cold or Allergies?" © 2005 Asthma and Allergy Foundation of America (www.aafa.org). All rights reserved. Reprinted with permission.

Diarrhea and vomiting also can occur but are more common in children. These symptoms are referred to as "flu-like symptoms." A lot of different illnesses, including the common cold, allergy symptoms, and asthma symptoms can sometimes be similar and confusing. Always consult with your doctor to make a proper diagnosis.

Emergency Flu Symptoms

There are some "emergency signs" that require immediate medical care. In children, emergency signs include:

- rapid breathing or difficulty breathing;

- blue skin color;

- not drinking enough fluids;

- not waking up or not being conscious;

- being irritable and inconsolable;

- flu-like symptoms seem to improve but return with worse fever and cough;

- fever with a rash.

For adults, emergency signs include:

- rapid breathing or difficulty breathing;

- pain in the chest or abdomen;

- sudden dizziness;

- confusion;

- severe or persistent vomiting.

> ♣ **It's A Fact!!**
> **Common Flu Symptoms**
>
> The flu usually starts suddenly and may include these symptoms:
>
> - Fever (often very high 101° F or above)
> - Headache
> - Extreme tiredness, chills
> - Constant cough
> - Sore throat
> - Runny or stuffy nose
> - Body aches in bones and/or muscles
>
> Source: © 2009 Asthma and Allergy Foundation of America.

How Does The Flu Spread?

The flu spreads in respiratory spraying from coughing and sneezing. It usually spreads from person to person, though occasionally someone could become infected by touching something with virus on it and touching their mouth or nose. Adults may be able to infect others one day before getting symptoms and up to seven days after getting sick. So it's possible to give the flu before you know you're sick, as well as while you are sick.

Prevention

The single best way to prevent the flu is to get a flu vaccine (a flu shot) each fall. Who should get a flu shot every year:

- adults 50 years or older;

- all children aged six–23 months;

- people of any age with chronic medical conditions (such as asthma, heart or lung disease, transplant recipients, or persons with HIV/AIDS);

- all women who will be pregnant during the influenza season;

- people in nursing homes;

- health-care workers involved in patient care;

- caregivers of people in high-risk groups mentioned above.

Also, a few antiviral drugs are approved for prevention of the flu. These are prescription medications, and a doctor should be consulted before they are used. In addition, there are some easy things you can do to prevent the spread of respiratory illnesses like the flu:

- Cover your nose/mouth with a cloth or tissue when you cough/sneeze—throw it away after use.

- Wash hands often with soap and water, especially after coughing/sneezing. If you don't have access to running water, use an alcohol-based hand cleanser.

☞ Remember!!
Diagnosing The Flu

There are tests that determine if you have the flu if tested within the first three days of illness. Also, a doctor's exam may be needed to tell whether you have an infection that is a complication of the flu.

Source: © 2009 Asthma and Allergy Foundation of America.

- Stay away from people who are sick.
- If you get the flu, stay home from work or school.
- Try not to touch your eyes, nose, or mouth. This is how germs often spread.

Treating The Flu

Antiviral Medications: Some antiviral drugs are approved for treatment of the flu. They are prescription medications, and a doctor should be consulted

---

♣ It's A Fact!!
"Swine" Flu (The H1N1 Strain)

Information from the U.S. Centers for Disease Control and Prevention (CDC) suggests that many of the signs and symptoms of swine flu are similar to those experienced by people with seasonal allergies. If your runny nose, itchy and watery eyes, sore throat, and other common allergy symptoms are combined with an unusually high fever (100 degrees or higher), chills, severe headache, or significant aches and pains, you could have some type influenza, including swine flu.

Swine flu symptoms are similar to typical flu symptoms and to common allergy effects as well. As an asthma and allergy patient, you must be particularly vigilant to avoid contact with people who might have any strain of influenza, including swine flu.

You can take several simple precautions to protect yourself and the members of your family from contracting influenza. The CDC recommends taking the following steps:

- Cover your nose and mouth with a tissue when you cough or sneeze.
- Wash your hands often with soap and water, especially after you cough or sneeze. Alcohol-based hand cleaners are also effective.
- Avoid touching your eyes, nose, or mouth.
- Try to avoid close contact with sick people.
- If you get sick with influenza, CDC recommends that you stay home from work or school and limit contact with others to keep from infecting them.

before the drugs are used. Antiviral treatment lasts for five days and must be started within two days of illness so if you get flu-like symptoms, seek medical care early on.

Other: If you get the flu, get plenty of rest, drink a lot of liquids, and avoid using alcohol and tobacco. Also, you can take medications to relieve the symptoms of the flu (but never give aspirin to children or teenagers who have flu-like symptoms, particularly fever).

If you think your allergy symptoms might be indicative of something more severe, including any strain of influenza, you should visit your primary care physician for a diagnosis or treatment recommendation. Further, if you become ill and experience any of the following warning signs, seek emergency medical care:

Emergency warning signs that need urgent medical attention for children include:

- Fast breathing or trouble breathing
- Bluish skin color
- Not drinking enough fluids
- Not waking up or not interacting
- Being so irritable that the child does not want to be held
- Flu-like symptoms improve but then return with fever and worse cough
- Fever with a rash

Emergency warning signs that need urgent medical attention for adults include:

- Difficulty breathing or shortness of breath
- Pain or pressure in the chest or abdomen
- Sudden dizziness
- Confusion
- Severe or persistent vomiting

For more information, including up-to-date statistical data on the swine flu situation in the United States, please visit http://www.cdc.gov/swineflu/.

Source: © 2009 Asthma and Allergy Foundation of America.

Flu/Cold Or Allergies?

Cough. Sneeze. Wheeze. You know the symptoms, but do you really know the cause? The similarities between symptoms of the flu/cold and nasal allergies (also called allergic rhinitis, indoor or outdoor allergies, seasonal allergies or hay-fever) can cause confusion. Worse, it can cause you to make the wrong diagnosis and treat with the wrong medications. And, if allergies are left untreated, it can cause more serious conditions like sinusitis or ear infections.

Learn about the difference in Table 34.1, and talk to your doctor about a complete medical exam to find out for sure.

Table 34.1. The Differences Between Symptoms Of Flu/Cold And Allergies

	Allergies	Flu/Cold
Symptoms	Allergies usually cause runny nose (**clear** discharge), stuffed nose, violent sneezing, wheezing, coughing, watery and itchy eyes.	Flu/cold usually includes runny nose (**yellow** discharge), aches and pains, sore and scratchy throat along with sneezing and coughing.
Fever	There is **no fever** with allergies.	If you have a **fever** it is almost certainly a flu/cold rather than allergies.
When	**Anytime** of the year: spring, summer, fall or winter.	Usually appear in **winter**, but are also possible in the fall, spring or summer.
Warning	Symptoms begin almost **immediately** after exposure to allergens.	Usually takes a **few days** for flu/cold symptoms to appear.
Duration	Symptoms last **a long time**, as long you are exposed to the allergen. If the allergen is present all year long, symptoms can be chronic.	Flu/cold symptoms should clear up within **a few days** to a week. Rarely lasts more than 10 days.

♣ It's A Fact!!
Viral Infections And Asthma

Respiratory infections, such as head or chest colds, are common ailments, and viruses are often the cause. Symptoms include a runny nose, a sore throat, and maybe a cough. Although they can make anyone feel miserable, do these infections affect people with asthma more severely? Interestingly, researchers have found scientific evidence to support two contradictory effects of respiratory viruses on asthma:

- Viral infections can make asthma symptoms worse.

- Viral infections may help protect children against asthma development later in life.

A review of a few medical studies may help explain these different conclusions. The authors of a study published in 2002 analyzed respiratory symptoms in couples among whom one partner had allergic asthma (which is influenced by family history) and the other did not. The researchers found no difference between the partners in frequency, severity, and duration of upper respiratory symptoms (in the head and throat). In those with allergic asthma, however, they found twice the frequency, increased severity, and longer duration of lower respiratory symptoms (in the lungs and airways). Studies such as these support the notion that viral respiratory infections (such as colds and bronchitis) are probably the most common cause of worsening asthma symptoms, accounting for at least 30 to 40 percent of asthma flare-ups in adults.

In contrast, a study of children and their siblings who had had non-respiratory viral infections (such as measles, mumps, or chickenpox) during the first year of life showed a small protective effect against asthma development. But when respiratory infections were singled out for analysis, scientists noticed an increase in asthma risk.

In another study, children at age three who had occasional upper respiratory infections showed a lower risk of asthma by age seven. But it was found that children who had lower respiratory infections were at significantly increased risk for asthma.

This study suggests that the effect of respiratory viruses on asthma development depends on numerous factors—for example, whether a virus affects the upper or lower respiratory tract, the frequency and severity of viral infections, a person's age when exposed to viruses, and family history of asthma.

In light of the medical research, viral respiratory infections clearly have the ability to worsen asthma symptoms in people who already have the disease. But claiming that they offer some protection against developing asthma is probably a conclusion that needs further research.

Flu/Colds

A flu/cold is commonly caused by a virus. You can get a flu/cold from another person that has that virus, even though you may be in good health. This happens when you breathe in germs or come in direct contact with the infected person. To prevent yourself from getting a flu/cold, get a flu shot every year, frequently wash your hands, use a disinfectant on your hands, and be careful when sneezing and coughing around others.

Allergies

Nasal allergies occur during exposure to an allergen, and your nasal cavity becomes irritated and inflamed. Unlike the flu/cold, allergies are not contagious. If you have a high temperature or an achy body, it is most likely a flu/cold rather than allergies. Common indoor and outdoor allergens include tree, grass, and weed pollen, dust mites, animal dander, mold, and cockroaches.

There is no cure for allergies, but there are prescription and over-the-counter medications treat allergy symptoms. For some people, allergy shots (immunotherapy), can help to reduce your sensitivity to allergens over time. Talk to your doctor about the best treatment plan for you.

✔ **Quick Tip**

Let a flu/cold run its course. Get rest, drink lots of fluids, and eat healthy foods. Over-the-counter medications, like an decongestant or a nasal sprays, can help relieve your symptoms, but they do not cure your cold—only time can do that.

Source: © 2005 Asthma and Allergy Foundation of America.

Chapter 35

Coughing: A Defense Mechanism And A Symptom

Is coughing normal or abnormal?

It is normal to cough occasionally. Excessive coughing or coughing that brings up blood or thick, discolored mucus is abnormal. Abnormal coughing can also leave you feeling exhausted or light-headed, cause chest or abdominal discomfort, or even cause you to "wet" yourself.

What causes cough?

Whether coughing is normal or abnormal, it has a purpose. Coughing is the body's way of keeping foreign matter from getting down into your lungs—like when you swallow a piece of food "the wrong way" and immediately cough it up. Coughing also helps to clear excessive mucus from your air passages. You may have excessive mucus in your air passages if you are a smoker, if you have a cold or other respiratory infection, or if your normal mucus-clearing mechanisms do not work properly. Even if your coughing is not productive, it is a signal that something is wrong and that you need to see your doctor.

About This Chapter: Text in this chapter is from "Information for Patients Complaining of Cough," © 2009 American College of Chest Physicians (www.chestnet.org). Reprinted with permission.

What is the cause if a person cannot stop coughing?

Doctors divide coughing into three different categories, based on how long the cough has gone on. They call these categories *acute* (for coughing of less than three weeks), *subacute* (for coughing of three to eight weeks), and *chronic* (for coughing of more than eight weeks).

Acute, Subacute, And Chronic Cough

- *Acute Cough (Less Than Three Weeks):* Most often, caused by a "common cold." It is usually worse for the first few days of a cold, then gradually goes away in one or two weeks, as you get over the cold.

- *Subacute Cough (Three to Eight Weeks):* Often, a cough that lingers after a cold or other respiratory tract infection is over. A subacute cough may eventually go away without treatment but may need to be treated by a doctor after its cause is diagnosed. An example of a subacute cough that requires treatment is one that persists after whooping cough.

- *Chronic Cough (More Than Eight Weeks):* Due to one or more of the conditions described in more detail below. The most common causes are upper airway cough syndrome (UACS), asthma, and gastroesophageal reflux disease (GERD). Chronic cough is also common in smokers.

What about the causes of chronic cough?

The most common causes are UACS, asthma, and GERD.

Common Causes Of Chronic Cough

- *Upper Airway Cough Syndrome (UACS):* UACS includes conditions that cause cough by affecting the nose, sinuses, or throat. They stimulate cough nerve endings by a combination of postnasal drip, irritation, or inflammation of the tissues. Upper respiratory tract infection, allergies,

♣ **It's A Fact!!**
How does the body know when to make you cough?

The body has a cough "trigger." Foreign matter or excessive mucus in your air passages irritates special nerve endings in your respiratory tract. When these nerve endings are irritated, they signal the body to cough.

and exposure to environmental irritants, such as dusts and gases, are the usual cause of UACS.

- *Asthma:* Asthma is a disease in which the air passages of the lungs are inflamed and narrowed. This happens in response to "triggers," such as allergens (pollen, dust mites, and many others), cold air, or infections. Airway narrowing and increased "twitchiness" (or responsiveness to a "trigger") can make the airway narrow and cause coughing.

- *Gastroesophageal Reflux Disease (GERD):* GERD is caused when stomach juice backs up from the stomach into the esophagus, the tube that carries food from your mouth and throat down into your stomach. Stomach juice contains acid and enzymes that help to digest the food you swallow. If it backs up (refluxes) into your throat, it can cause burning pain and cause you to cough. The burning pain is sometimes called "heartburn." However, most people who have chronic cough from GERD do not have heartburn. This is called "silent GERD."

What about smoking as a cause of cough?

"Smoker's cough" is often due to a lung disease called chronic bronchitis, a disease most commonly caused by cigarette smoking. Irritation from the smoke causes increased mucus production and inflammation of the large air passages of the lungs. Most smokers do not seek medical attention for this cough, because they assume it is from smoking. Sometimes, however, a smoker is coughing from another cause. Just as in nonsmokers, the cough could be from UACS, asthma, or GERD, but it also could be a warning of an even more serious disorder, like lung cancer.

♣ It's A Fact!!

If you are coughing from cigarette smoking and chronic bronchitis, will the cough go away if you stop smoking? Typically, it will, but it can take four weeks to as long as a few months. If the cough seems different from your usual "smoker's cough," or if it persists despite stopping smoking for a month or longer, it definitely should be checked out by your doctor.

What other conditions cause chronic cough?

There are many other causes, but only a few occur often enough to discuss in this chapter. The following are some of the more frequent causes:

• Nonasthmatic eosinophilic bronchitis has some similarities to asthma, but its only significant symptom is cough. It is seen more frequently in countries outside the United States but should be considered, especially if UACS, asthma, GERD, and cigarette smoking have been eliminated as causes of the coughing.

• An important cause of chronic cough is related to a class of medication often used to treat high blood pressure or heart problems. This group of drugs is known as angiotensin-converting enzyme inhibitors, or ACE inhibitors. They can produce a very annoying cough, often associated with throat irritation. The cough may not occur until a person has been on the medication for many months. It will always go away within days to weeks once the medication is stopped.

• Bronchiectasis is a disease in which parts of the lower air passages are damaged, dilated, and prone to recurrent infection. It can cause a cough that persists after a respiratory tract infection, lung cancer, and inflammatory or scarring diseases of the lungs.

• Chronic cough can also be due to heart failure. There are many uncommon causes of chronic cough, too many to list here. You and your doctor can look them up in this guideline: Diagnosis and Management of Cough: ACCP Evidence-Based Clinical Practice Guidelines. *CHEST* 2006; 129(suppl):1s-292s.

Can you have more than one cause of chronic cough at the same time?

Absolutely. In fact, it is common for two causes to be present simultaneously, and, sometimes, even three or more will be present.

Is it important to determine the specific cause(s) of a chronic cough?

Yes. Chronic coughing can be more than annoying. It can lead to complications, such as fatigue, sweating, and even broken ribs from really hard coughing. It can make you worry that something may be seriously wrong with your health. The best way to get rid of your cough and these complications is to treat the underlying cause(s).

What is the best way for a doctor to determine the cause(s) of a cough?

A combination of selected tests and targeted treatments allow the specific cause(s) of a chronic cough to be determined in the vast majority of cases. A lung specialist (pulmonologist) should be able to determine the cause(s) in about 90 percent of cases. When a cause cannot be determined, a referral and visit to a cough specialist (pulmonologist with particular expertise in cough) will usually result in an answer in the majority of these more difficult cases.

Does treatment for chronic cough usually work?

Yes. In over 90 percent of cases, the cough will be greatly improved or disappear entirely with treatment. The key is to use the correct medications at the right dose for each cause of the cough. The length of treatment is also very important. Whether the cause is a UACS, asthma, GERD, or one of the less common causes, it is not unusual for treatment to take weeks, even months, to be completely successful. This is particularly true for GERD.

What tests are done to diagnose the cause(s) of chronic cough?

A chest x-ray is recommended for all patients with chronic cough. If the x-ray has negative results, your doctor may decide not to order additional tests until he or she has seen your response to therapy. If you do not respond to treatment as expected, your doctor may also order a variety of other tests. These may include breathing tests, blood studies, sputum studies, other x-rays (such as those of the sinuses), barium swallow, and other gastrointestinal tests, such as 24-hour monitoring of the function of the esophagus, a CAT scan of the lungs, or a bronchoscopy.

Breathing tests are done primarily to see if you might have asthma as a cause of cough. If the initial test shows you have normal lung function, then a test may be done to detect overactivity of the air passages of the lungs. This test is called a bronchoprovocation challenge, and it should be done before asthma is ruled out as the cause of your cough. This test involves breathing a medication (most often one called *methacholine*). You breathe this medication in, and then the breathing test is repeated. If you have asthma, your lung function will decrease at least 20 percent for a short period of time. The decrease can usually be reversed quickly by inhaling a common asthma medication.

A bronchoscopy involves putting a thin, flexible tube, containing a tiny video camera, through the nose or mouth, down into the air passages of the lungs. This is a relatively painless and safe test when done by a lung specialist. This test can detect tumors, infections, foreign bodies, or other abnormalities of the lower air passages that could be causing chronic cough. It is only needed in a small number of patients who usually have a significant abnormality on the initial chest x-ray. When the initial chest x-ray has normal results, a bronchoscopy result will also typically be normal, and, therefore, it should not be one of the first tests done. However, later in the workup, if the common causes have been eliminated, a bronchoscopy test should be done, because, occasionally, an uncommon cause of the chronic cough is discovered by this test.

Chapter 36

Gastroesophageal Reflux Disease (GERD) And Asthma

What is GERD?

Gastroesophageal reflux disease (GERD) is a more serious form of gastroesophageal reflux (GER), which is common. GER occurs when the lower esophageal sphincter (LES) opens spontaneously, for varying periods of time, or does not close properly and stomach contents rise up into the esophagus. GER is also called acid reflux or acid regurgitation, because digestive juices—called acids—rise up with the food. The esophagus is the tube that carries food from the mouth to the stomach. The LES is a ring of muscle at the bottom of the esophagus that acts like a valve between the esophagus and stomach.

When acid reflux occurs, food or fluid can be tasted in the back of the mouth. When refluxed stomach acid touches the lining of the esophagus it may cause a burning sensation in the chest or throat called heartburn or acid indigestion. Occasional GER is common and does not necessarily mean one has GERD. Persistent reflux that occurs more than twice a week is considered GERD, and it can eventually lead to more serious health problems. People of all ages can have GERD.

About This Chapter: Text in this chapter is from "Heartburn, Gastroesophageal Reflux (GER), and Gastroesophageal Reflux Disease (GERD)," The National Digestive Diseases Information Clearinghouse (NDDIC), NIH Publication No. 07–0882, May 2007.

What are the symptoms of GERD?

The main symptom of GERD in adults is frequent heartburn, also called acid indigestion—burning-type pain in the lower part of the mid-chest, behind the breast bone, and in the mid-abdomen. Most children under 12 years with GERD, and some adults, have GERD without heartburn. Instead, they may experience a dry cough, asthma symptoms, or trouble swallowing.

What causes GERD?

The reason some people develop GERD is still unclear. However, research shows that in people with GERD, the LES relaxes while the rest of the esophagus is working. Anatomical abnormalities such as a hiatal hernia may also contribute to GERD. A hiatal hernia occurs when the upper part of the stomach and the LES move above the diaphragm, the muscle wall that separates the stomach from the chest. Normally, the diaphragm helps the LES keep acid from rising up into the esophagus. When a hiatal hernia is present, acid reflux can occur more easily. A hiatal hernia can occur in people of any age and is most often a normal finding in otherwise healthy people over age 50. Most of the time, a hiatal hernia produces no symptoms.

Other factors that may contribute to GERD include the following:

- Obesity

- Pregnancy

- Smoking

What is GERD in children?

Distinguishing between normal, physiologic reflux and GERD in children is important. Most infants with GER are happy and healthy even if they frequently spit up or vomit, and babies usually outgrow GER by their first birthday. Reflux that continues past one year

> **☞ Remember!!**
>
> Common foods that can worsen reflux symptoms include the following:
>
> - Citrus fruits
>
> - Chocolate
>
> - Drinks with caffeine or alcohol
>
> - Fatty and fried foods
>
> - Garlic and onions
>
> - Mint flavorings
>
> - Spicy foods
>
> - Tomato-based foods, like spaghetti sauce, salsa, chili, and pizza

of age may be GERD. Studies show GERD is common and may be overlooked in infants and children. For example, GERD can present as repeated regurgitation, nausea, heartburn, coughing, laryngitis, or respiratory problems like wheezing, asthma, or pneumonia. Infants and young children may demonstrate irritability or arching of the back, often during or immediately after feedings. Infants with GERD may refuse to feed and experience poor growth.

Parents should talk with their child's health care provider if reflux-related symptoms occur regularly and cause the child discomfort. The health care provider may recommend simple strategies for avoiding reflux, such as burping the infant several times during feeding or keeping the infant in an upright position for 30 minutes after feeding. If the child is older, the health care provider may recommend that the child eat small, frequent meals and avoid the following foods:

- Sodas that contain caffeine
- Chocolate
- Peppermint
- Spicy foods
- Acidic foods like oranges, tomatoes, and pizza
- Fried and fatty foods

Avoiding food two to three hours before bed may also help. The health care provider may recommend raising the head of a child's bed with wood blocks secured under the bedposts. Just using extra pillows will not help. If these changes do not work, the health care provider may prescribe medicine for the child. In rare cases, a child may need surgery.

How is GERD treated?

See your health care provider if you have had symptoms of GERD and have been using antacids or other over-the-counter reflux medications for more than two weeks. Your health care provider may refer you to a gastroenterologist, a doctor who treats diseases of the stomach and intestines. Depending on the severity of your GERD, treatment may involve one or more of the following lifestyle changes, medications, or surgery.

Lifestyle Changes

- If you smoke, stop

- Avoid foods and beverages that worsen symptoms

- Lose weight if needed

- Eat small, frequent meals

- Wear loose-fitting clothes

- Avoid lying down for three hours after a meal

- Raise the head of your bed six to eight inches by securing wood blocks under the bedposts. Just using extra pillows will not help.

What medications are used to treat GERD?

Your health care provider may recommend over-the-counter antacids or medications that stop acid production or help the muscles that empty your stomach. You can buy many of these medications without a prescription. However, see your health care provider before starting or adding a medication.

Antacids: Antacids, such as Alka-Seltzer, Maalox, Mylanta, Rolaids, and Riopan, are usually the first drugs recommended to relieve heartburn and other mild GERD symptoms. Many brands on the market use different combinations of three basic salts—magnesium, calcium, and aluminum—with hydroxide or bicarbonate ions to neutralize the acid in your stomach. Antacids, however, can have side effects. Magnesium salt can lead to diarrhea, and aluminum salt may cause constipation. Aluminum and magnesium salts are often combined in a single product to balance these effects.

Calcium Carbonate Antacids: Calcium carbonate antacids, such as Tums, Titralac, and Alka-2, can also be a supplemental source of calcium. They can cause constipation as well.

Foaming Agents: Foaming agents, such as Gaviscon, work by covering your stomach contents with foam to prevent reflux.

H2 Blockers: H2 blockers, such as cimetidine (Tagamet HB), famotidine (Pepcid AC), nizatidine (Axid AR), and ranitidine (Zantac 75), decrease acid production. They are available in prescription strength and over-the-counter strength. These drugs provide short-term relief and are effective for about half of those who have GERD symptoms.

Proton Pump Inhibitors: Proton pump inhibitors include omeprazole (Prilosec, Zegerid), lansoprazole (Prevacid), pantoprazole (Protonix), rabeprazole (Aciphex), and esomeprazole (Nexium), which are available by prescription. Prilosec is also available in over-the-counter strength. Proton pump inhibitors are more effective than H2 blockers and can relieve symptoms and heal the esophageal lining in almost everyone who has GERD.

Prokinetics: Prokinetics help strengthen the LES and make the stomach empty faster. This group includes bethanechol (Urecholine) and metoclopramide (Reglan). Metoclopramide also improves muscle action in the digestive tract. Prokinetics have frequent side effects that limit their usefulness—fatigue, sleepiness, depression, anxiety, and problems with physical movement.

Because drugs work in different ways, combinations of medications may help control symptoms. People who get heartburn after eating may take both antacids and H2 blockers. The antacids work first to neutralize the acid in the stomach, and then the H2 blockers act on acid production. By the time the antacid stops working, the H2 blocker will have stopped acid production. Your health care provider is the best source of information about how to use medications for GERD.

What if GERD symptoms persist?

If your symptoms do not improve with lifestyle changes or medications, you may need additional tests.

Barium Swallow Radiograph: Barium swallow radiograph uses x-rays to help spot abnormalities such as a hiatal hernia and other structural or anatomical problems of the esophagus. With this test, you drink a solution and then x-rays are taken. The test will not detect mild irritation, although strictures—narrowing of the esophagus—and ulcers can be observed.

Upper Endoscopy: Upper endoscopy is more accurate than a barium swallow radiograph and may be performed in a hospital or a doctor's office. The doctor may spray your throat to numb it and then, after lightly sedating you, will slide a thin, flexible plastic tube with a light and lens on the end called an endoscope down your throat. Acting as a tiny camera, the endoscope allows the doctor to see the surface of the esophagus and search for abnormalities. If you have had moderate to severe symptoms and this procedure reveals injury to the esophagus, usually no other tests are needed to confirm GERD.

The doctor also may perform a biopsy. Tiny tweezers, called forceps, are passed through the endoscope and allow the doctor to remove small pieces of tissue from your esophagus. The tissue is then viewed with a microscope to look for damage caused by acid reflux and to rule out other problems if infection or abnormal growths are not found.

pH Monitoring Examination: pH monitoring examination involves the doctor either inserting a small tube into the esophagus or clipping a tiny device to the esophagus that will stay there for 24 to 48 hours. While you go about your normal activities, the device measures when and how much acid comes up into your esophagus. This test can be useful if combined with a carefully completed diary—recording when, what, and amounts the person eats—which allows the doctor to see correlations between symptoms and reflux episodes. The procedure is sometimes helpful in detecting whether respiratory symptoms, including wheezing and coughing, are triggered by reflux.

A completely accurate diagnostic test for GERD does not exist, and tests have not consistently shown that acid exposure to the lower esophagus directly correlates with damage to the lining.

When is surgery considered as a treatment option?

Surgery is an option when medicine and lifestyle changes do not help to manage GERD symptoms. Surgery may also be a reasonable alternative to a lifetime of drugs and discomfort.

Fundoplication: Fundoplication is the standard surgical treatment for GERD. Usually a specific type of this procedure, called *Nissen fundoplication*, is performed. During the Nissen fundoplication, the upper part of the stomach is wrapped around the LES to strengthen the sphincter, prevent acid reflux, and repair a hiatal hernia.

The Nissen fundoplication may be performed using a laparoscope, an instrument that is inserted through tiny incisions in the abdomen. The doctor then uses small instruments that hold a camera to look at the abdomen and pelvis. When performed by experienced surgeons, laparoscopic fundoplication is safe and effective in people of all ages, including infants. The procedure is reported to have the same results as the standard fundoplication, and people can leave the hospital in one to three days and return to work in two to three weeks.

☞ Remember!!
Points To Remember

- Frequent heartburn, also called acid indigestion, is the most common symptom of GERD in adults. Anyone experiencing heartburn twice a week or more may have GERD.

- You can have GERD without having heartburn. Your symptoms could include a dry cough, asthma symptoms, or trouble swallowing.

- If you have been using antacids for more than two weeks, it is time to see your health care provider. Most doctors can treat GERD. Your health care provider may refer you to a gastroenterologist, a doctor who treats diseases of the stomach and intestines.

- Health care providers usually recommend lifestyle and dietary changes to relieve symptoms of GERD. Many people with GERD also need medication. Surgery may be considered as a treatment option.

- Most infants with GER are healthy even though they may frequently spit up or vomit. Most infants outgrow GER by their first birthday. Reflux that continues past one year of age may be GERD.

- The persistence of GER along with other symptoms—arching and irritability in infants, or abdominal and chest pain in older children—is GERD. GERD is the outcome of frequent and persistent GER in infants and children and may cause repeated vomiting, coughing, and respiratory problems.

Endoscopic techniques used to treat chronic heartburn include the Bard EndoCinch system, NDO Plicator, and the Stretta system. These techniques require the use of an endoscope to perform the anti-reflux operation. The EndoCinch and NDO Plicator systems involve putting stitches in the LES to create pleats that help strengthen the muscle. The Stretta system uses electrodes to create tiny burns on the LES. When the burns heal, the scar tissue helps toughen the muscle. The long-term effects of these three procedures are unknown.

What are the long-term complications of GERD?

Chronic GERD that is untreated can cause serious complications. Inflammation of the esophagus from refluxed stomach acid can damage the lining and cause bleeding or ulcers—also called esophagitis. Scars from tissue damage can lead to strictures—narrowing of the esophagus—that make swallowing difficult. Some people develop Barrett's esophagus, in which cells in the esophageal lining take on an abnormal shape and color. Over time, the cells can lead to esophageal cancer, which is often fatal. Persons with GERD and its complications should be monitored closely by a physician.

Studies have shown that GERD may worsen or contribute to asthma, chronic cough, and pulmonary fibrosis.

Hope Through Research

The reasons certain people develop GERD and others do not remain unknown. Several factors may be involved, and research is under way to explore risk factors for developing GERD and the role of GERD in other conditions such as asthma and laryngitis.

Chapter 37

Osteoporosis: Risks For People With Asthma

What Is Osteoporosis?

Osteoporosis is a serious condition in which bones become thin, brittle and easily broken. The National Osteoporosis Foundation (NOF) estimates that more than 44 million Americans have osteoporosis or low bone density placing them at risk for osteoporosis. This represents 55 percent of people aged 50 and older in the United States.

While the majority (80 percent) of persons affected by osteoporosis are women, one in eight men also suffers from the disease. This rate is expected to increase as men live longer. Similarly, while osteoporosis is more prevalent in Caucasian and Asian populations, African Americans and Latinos are also at significant risk of developing the disease. Osteoporosis is called the "silent disease" because people do not know that they have osteoporosis until their bones become so weak that a sudden strain, bump, a fall, or even a sneeze can cause a fracture.

The most common fractures associated with osteoporosis include wrist, vertebral and hip fractures. It is estimated that half of all women and 20 percent of all men will have an osteoporotic fracture in their lifetime. In the

About This Chapter: The information in this chapter, from "What Is Osteoporosis," "Asthma and Osteoporosis," "Calcium and Vitamin D," and "Exercise," is reprinted with permission from New Jersey Department of Health and Senior Services Division of Aging and Community Services, © 2009.

♣ It's A Fact!!

The disability associated with osteoporosis-related fractures places heavy demands on the health care system. The estimated national direct expenditures (hospitals and nursing homes) for osteoporotic and associated fractures was $13.8 billion in 1995 ($38 million each day) and the cost is rising.

The outlook for persons experiencing a hip fracture is particularly alarming:

- 20 percent of hip fracture patients may require long-term nursing home care.

- 50 percent never regain their ability to walk independently, and up to 20 percent die within one year due to complications of the fracture or accompanying surgery.

- Approximately 33 percent of people are totally dependent on others for their care following hip fracture.

United States, 300,000 hip fractures occur each year in persons age 65 and older. The majority of these hip fractures are associated with a fall in an individual with osteoporosis.

Osteoporosis is a pediatric disease with geriatric consequences. Peak bone mass is built during our first three decades. Failure to build strong bones during childhood and adolescent years manifests in fractures later in life.

The good news is that osteoporosis is both preventable and treatable. Steps can be taken at any age to prevent or minimize the effect of osteoporosis.

Asthma and Osteoporosis

The Asthma-Osteoporosis Connection: Millions of men, women, and children suffering from arthritis, asthma, or other diseases take corticosteroids, often resulting in the development of osteoporosis. Powerful anti-inflammatory drugs such as prednisone and cortisone greatly increase the risk of developing osteoporosis, a bone-thinning disease that leads to painful fractures, loss of height and independence, and can even lead to death. Check with your health care provider or pharmacist if you are taking asthma, arthritis, anti-inflammatory or anti-convulsant drugs.

Asthma And Bone Loss: Asthma affects between 12 and 14 million Americans, more than four million of whom are under the age of 18. Asthma is becoming more common, with African Americans especially at risk. People with asthma are at increased risk for osteoporosis, especially in the spine. Anti-inflammatory medications taken by mouth decrease calcium absorbed from food, increase calcium loss from the kidneys, and decrease bone formation. Corticosteroids also interfere with the production of sex hormones in both women and men, contributing to bone loss and causing muscle weakness, both of which can increase the risk of falling.

Asthma medication can increase risk of osteoporosis. People with asthma who are treated with 40 to 60 mg per day of oral corticosteroids for long periods of time are most likely to experience bone loss. Even those patients taking 10 mg per day are likely to experience some bone loss over time. Bone loss increases with increased glucocorticoid doses and prolonged use.

Asthmatics who use corticosteroids to manage their asthma are at significant risk for bone loss and should ask their doctor about a bone density test to measure their current bone mass and to diagnose osteoporosis before fractures occur.

Asthma And Osteoporosis Medications: Maintaining appropriate hormone levels of estrogen in women and testosterone in men will help maintain optimal bone health. At menopause, estrogen replacement therapy (ERT) or hormone replacement therapy (HRT) may effectively prevent the bone loss and osteoporosis resulting from corticosteroid use. Other medications to stop bone loss include Fosamax (alendronate), Miacalcin (calcitonin), Actonel (risedronate), and Evista (raloxifene).

Calcium And Asthma: Many asthma sufferers think that milk and dairy products trigger asthmatic attacks. This frequently results in the avoidance of dairy products, which is especially damaging for asthmatic children and adolescents who need calcium to build bone.

Exercise And Asthma: Physical exercise can trigger an asthma attack and many people with asthma avoid weight-bearing physical activities that can strengthen bone. Weight-bearing exercises that work the body against gravity, such as walking, racquet sports, basketball, volleyball, aerobics, dancing or weight-training can improve bone health. Talk to your health care provider or ask for a referral to physical therapist. Consult a physical therapist about the best types of exercise before beginning an exercise program.

Calcium And Vitamin D

To build strong bones, make sure you get enough calcium at every age.

Make sure you're taking enough calcium in your daily diet. The first choice for adequate calcium intake is from food. You need at least enough calcium to equal three to four eight-ounce glasses of milk each day. A variety of calcium-rich foods can provide you with the needed calcium.

- Make it a habit, take your calcium at the same times each day, such as when you finish meals or brush your teeth.

- Remember to eat foods with calcium several times throughout the day; your body uses calcium best when it can absorb it in small doses.

- Vitamin D helps build strong bones, you need 400-800 International Units of vitamin D each day.

- Calcium plays an important role in keeping bones strong, but calcium alone cannot prevent or cure osteoporosis.

☞ **Remember!!**

Osteoporosis is preventable and treatable.

Preventing Osteoporosis: The key to preventing osteoporosis is to eat calcium-rich foods and increase physical activity by doing weight-bearing or resistance exercises to build bone mass.

Your risk of developing osteoporosis depends on the amount of bone mass built through age 35, when most people reach their peak bone mass.

Source: The information in this box, from "Prevention," is reprinted with permission from New Jersey Department of Health and Senior Services Division of Aging and Community Services, © 2009.

✔ Quick Tip
YOU Can Take Steps To Build Peak Bone Mass

- Get plenty of calcium and physical activity early in life.

- Maintain your bone mass as you get older by eating foods high in calcium and vitamin D.

- Do weight-bearing or resistance activities.

- Live a healthy lifestyle—exercise regularly, limit alcohol, and avoid smoking.

- Speak with your doctor about specific steps to take to help keep your bones strong, including medications you can take to prevent the disease.

Diet And Nutrition: Dairy products and other foods high in calcium and vitamin D will help keep your bones strong. To build strong bones, make sure you get enough calcium at every age.

Exercise can help prevent osteoporosis. If you already have osteoporosis, exercise can help maintain bone strength.

Good News: If you have a diagnosis of osteoporosis, there are treatments to stop bone loss and, in some cases, you can increase bone strength.

Source: The information in this box, from "Prevention," is reprinted with permission from New Jersey Department of Health and Senior Services Division of Aging and Community Services, © 2009.

- If you have osteoporosis, proper nutrition and adequate calcium can help. Exercise can help, too.

Calcium To Prevent Bone Loss: Calcium and vitamin D in your diet protects the calcium in your bones. If you are not getting enough calcium, your bones become your body's emergency supply of calcium. When this happens, your bones become weak and break easily.

Many women consume less than half of the daily recommended amount of calcium. Calcium alone cannot prevent or cure osteoporosis, but it is an important part of preventing osteoporosis.

Foods Rich In Calcium And Vitamin D: Vitamin D plays a major role in calcium absorption and bone health. Vitamin D allows calcium to leave the intestine and enter the bloodstream. Vitamin D can be found in D-fortified dairy products, egg yolks, saltwater fish and liver. Vitamin D is manufactured in the skin following direct exposure to sunlight. About 10 to 15 minutes on your hands, arms and face two or three times a week meets the body's need for vitamin D. Since sunscreen diminishes the body's ability to manufacture Vitamin D, spend your first 10 to 15 minutes without sunscreen, then be sure to put on sunscreen for the remainder of your time outdoors. Remember, sunlight helps build strong bones.

Table 37.1. Daily Recommendation—How Much Calcium Does Your Body Need Each Day?

Children	Calcium
1–3 years	500 mg/day
4–8 years	800 mg/day
9–18 years	1,300 mg/day
Adults	**Calcium**
19–50	1,000 mg/day
51 and older	1,200 mg/day

Calcium Supplements: If you don't think you're getting enough calcium from your diet, talk to your health care provider or with a registered dietitian to learn about other foods that are high in calcium and bone-building nutrients. When necessary, supplements may also play a role in bone health. Speak with your physician or a pharmacist about your supplement options. Your body's supply of calcium needs to be replenished—take your calcium at various times throughout the day. Calcium carbonate (e.g., Tums or Oscal), contains the highest percent of calcium, is the least expensive and most widely used form of supplement. It is best absorbed if taken with food or right after eating and can cause gas or bowel problems.

• Calcium citrate (e.g., Citracal) is often added to breakfast products and juice. It's easier to absorb, but it contains the lowest amount of calcium and it is usually the most costly.

• Calcium phosphate (e.g., Posture) is easily absorbed and does not have to be taken with food, but has excessive phosphorus.

• Calcium lactate—avoid this form if dairy intolerant.

- Calcium gluconate requires many pills to get recommended minimum dose of calcium.

- Dolomite, bone meal may be contaminated with lead, so should be avoided.

Vitamin D: Vitamin D plays a major role in calcium absorption and bone health. Vitamin D_3 is manufactured in the skin following direct exposure to sunlight; however, there are many different factors that affect a person's ability to make adequate amounts of Vitamin D. Vitamin D is critical for health, especially for bone health. Vitamin D is a term used to name several forms of related compounds. All are fat-soluble and act to control calcium metabolism. Vitamin D is vital to absorption of calcium. But the way in which Vitamin D works is complicated. The various parts of Vitamin D metabolism happen throughout the body.

As little as 10 minutes of sunshine can make Vitamin D_3 in the skin. But in New Jersey, the angle of the sun is only in the right place from about the end of April through the middle of October. You need to sit in the sun with your skin exposed without sunscreen, of course. In the winter in the northeast, when the sun is too low, a dietary intake of Vitamin D becomes the sole source during those months. Vitamin D_3 either consumed in the diet or made in the skin is stored in the liver.

Food Sources: Vitamin D can be obtained from fortified milk, egg yolks, saltwater fish and liver. Some foods may be fortified with Vitamin D, including cereals, breakfast bars and milk alternatives, or supplements.

Supplements: Usually Vitamin D is supplied in tablets in the D_3 form, known as cholecalciferol.

♣ It's A Fact!!

According to NOF recommendations, adults under age 50 need 400–800 IU of vitamin D_3 daily, and adults age 50 and older need 800–1,000 IU of vitamin D_3 daily. Vitamin D_3 is the form of Vitamin D that best supports bone health.

Exercise

Exercise can help prevent osteoporosis. If you already have osteoporosis, exercise can help maintain bone strength.

Osteoporosis Exercise Guidelines

- Check with your physician concerning any restrictions you may have before beginning an exercise program.

- Avoid any exercise that causes or increases pain.

- Stop exercising if you feel dizzy or short of breath.

- Never hold your breath while exercising.

- Make sure to keep your body in alignment when performing all exercises.

- Avoid exercises that involve forward bending of your spine (i.e., toe touches, sit-ups). These exercises can increase the incidence of vertebral fractures.

- Avoid exercises that involve excessive twisting (i.e., windmill toe touches). This puts too much force on your spine.

- Do resistance exercises. Free weights, exercise machines, and resistance bands are examples of this type of exercise. Strive to do one set of eight to ten repetitions of each resistance exercise. For a more challenging program, progress to three sets of eight to ten repetitions.

- When using weights, rest one to two minutes between sets of exercises.

- When using weights, start with one-pound weights, then gradually increase the amount of weight. Too much weight can be harmful.

- Wear shoes with good support and cushioning while exercising. Replace shoes when cushioning begins to wear out.

Increase Your Exercise: Physical activity throughout life helps develop and maintain strong bones and decrease bone loss. Persons age 35 and older should consult their physician before beginning an exercise program. Your health care provider can make a referral to a physical therapist. Before you exercise, consult a physical therapist about the best types of exercise.

A complete osteoporosis exercise program should include weight-bearing, resistance, postural, and balance exercises. It is important to check with your physician or physical therapist before starting any exercise program.

Weight-bearing exercises use the weight of the body to work against gravity and are recommended for all ages. Your bones respond to this force by growing stronger. Walking, jogging, dancing, hiking, stair climbing, and aerobic exercises are all examples of weight-bearing exercises. The goal is to work up to 45 minutes or more per session. Perform these exercises at least three to five times per week. (Bike riding and swimming, although good exercises, are not weight bearing exercises).

Resistance exercises generate muscle tension on the bones and are recommended for everyone after the age of 14. Resistance exercise strengthens the muscles and stimulates the bones to grow stronger. Free weights, exercise machines and resistance bands are examples of this type of exercise. Start exercising without weights. Begin with one set of 8 to 10 repetitions of each exercise increasing gradually to three sets. When that becomes easy, add one lb. of weight at a time. These exercises should be done two to three times a week but not on consecutive days.

Postural exercises decrease harmful stress on the back. By performing these exercises, you can reduce your risk of spinal fractures and the rounded shoulders commonly seen with osteoporosis. These exercises should be performed throughout the day to reinforce good posture.

Balance exercises help maintain equilibrium and reduce the risk of falling. These exercises should be performed daily.

✔ Quick Tip

If you have osteoporosis, check with your doctor before doing high impact activities like jogging or high-impact aerobics. These exercises jar the spine and might increase the risk of spinal fractures.

Exercise And The Role Of The Physical Therapist: A physical therapist can design an exercise program that is safe and appropriate for both prevention and treatment of osteoporosis. Physical therapists are trained to teach proper ways to perform daily activities to reduce fracture risk. Talk to your physician about referral to a physical therapist.

Many individuals with osteoporosis will have postural changes, muscle, and soft tissue tightness that requires the hands-on treatment of a physical therapist.

Chapter 38

Rhinitis And Sinusitis

Almost everyone knows what it feels like to have a runny, stuffed-up nose at times. Often these symptoms are accompanied by a headache in the area around the eyes, nose and temples. People with allergies are especially prone to these symptoms. They are signs of rhinitis and sinusitis, two very common medical problems. It is estimated that up to 40 million American adults and children have one or both of these conditions.

Although not life-threatening, rhinitis and sinusitis can make you miserable. At their worst, they can keep you from functioning normally, and may lead to life-threatening complications. Fortunately, there are things you can do to prevent these problems. And effective treatments exist when these symptoms do arise. If you have allergies, you are more likely to develop rhinitis or sinusitis than are persons without allergies. This makes it even more important to keep your allergies under control and to prevent rhinitis and sinusitis from occurring.

What is rhinitis?

The word *rhinitis* means simply "inflammation of the nose." The nose normally produces a fluid called mucus. This fluid is normally thin and clear. It helps to keep dust, debris, and allergens out of the lungs. Mucus traps particles like dust and pollen as well as bacteria and viruses.

Normally, mucus drains down the back of the throat, but you're not aware of it due to its relatively small amount and thin consistency. But when the nose becomes irritated, it may produce more mucus, which becomes thick and pale yellow. The mucus may begin to flow from the front of the nose as well as the back. Substances in the mucus may irritate the back of the throat and cause coughing. This increased mucus draining down the throat is called *postnasal drip*.

What causes rhinitis?

Rhinitis may be caused by irritants or allergens (substances that provoke an allergic response). In response to these substances, the cells of the body release *histamine* and other chemical mediators. These are the substances that cause the symptoms of allergic rhinitis—sneezing, runny nose, and itching, watery eyes.

In many people, rhinitis is a temporary condition that clears up on its own after a few days. In others, especially those with allergies, rhinitis is a chronic problem—one that is nearly always present or that recurs often. Rhinitis is often classified into several types:

Allergic Rhinitis: Rhinitis caused by an allergic reaction may be either *seasonal*—occurring only at certain times of the year—or *perennial*—occurring year round. Seasonal allergic rhinitis is sometimes called "hay fever." It is an allergic reaction to pollen from trees and grasses. Ragweed pollen is another frequent culprit causing hay fever. This type of rhinitis occurs mainly in the spring and fall, when these pollens from trees, grasses and weeds are in the air.

Perennial allergic rhinitis is caused by allergies to substances that are present year round. The chief causes of this type of rhinitis are allergies to dust mites, mold, animal dander, and cockroach debris.

Nonallergic Rhinitis: Sometimes perennial rhinitis is not caused by allergic triggers. It may be caused by overuse of topical nose sprays, hormonal changes, structural abnormalities of the nose (such as septal deviation), and occasionally by medications. Often, the cause of this type of rhinitis is not well understood, but it is commonly present in patients with asthma. Its symptoms are similar to those produced by allergy.

Infectious Rhinitis: Perhaps the most common form of rhinitis, infectious rhinitis is also known as the common cold. It is caused by infection with a cold virus that takes up residence in the mucous membranes of the nose and sinus cavities.

It can be hard to tell the difference between allergies and the common cold. There are more than a hundred strains of cold viruses. Each tends to become widespread at certain times of the year, which is why you may mistake a cold for a seasonal allergy.

How is rhinitis treated?

Most cases of rhinitis go away once the source of irritation is gone. In the meantime, decongestants can help to relieve a stuffy nose. Be very careful, however, with the use of over-the-counter decongestant nasal sprays. Overuse of these products can actually make your stuffy nose worse. If used chronically and then stopped, after the effects of these products wear off, the tissue inside the nose and sinuses tends to become swollen. This can prompt you to use more of the medication, after which these tissues swell even more. A vicious cycle can begin if you keep using the product. As your body adjusts to the chronic medication, you need more of the medication more often to relieve the side effects. At first you may get relief, but in the long run the symptoms are worse. You then try to relieve the symptoms with more medication, which in turn worsens the side effects, and so on. All the while the underlying cause of your stuffy nose is not being treated.

Perhaps the most widely used type of medication used to control the symptoms of rhinitis are the *antihistamines*. These medications counteract the affects of histamine, the naturally occurring chemical that causes allergy symptoms. The chief side effect of antihistamines is drowsiness. A number of new antihistamines have been developed that do not cause drowsiness in most people. These medications are available with a doctor's prescription. Cromolyn nose spray, available over the counter, may be helpful for allergic rhinitis and causes essentially no side effects. The most effective medications for allergic rhinitis are the prescription corticosteroid nose sprays that reduce allergic inflammation, usually without causing systemic side effects.

What is sinusitis?

Sinusitis is an infection or inflammation of the sinuses. A *sinus* is simply a hollow space. There are many sinuses in the body, including four pairs inside the skull. These are called the *paranasal sinuses*. They serve to lighten the skull and give resonance to the voice.

The paranasal sinuses are lined with the same kind of tissue that lines the inside of the nose. The same things that can cause swelling in the nose—such as allergies or infection—can also affect the sinuses. When the tissue inside the sinuses becomes inflamed, mucus discharge is increased. Over time, air trapped inside the swollen sinuses can create painful pressure inside the head. This is what is known as a "sinus headache."

What causes sinusitis?

Most cases of sinusitis are caused by infection with a virus. If the sinuses remain blocked for a long time, though, a secondary infection may result. This secondary infection is caused by bacteria that are normally present within the respiratory tract. These bacteria multiply and cause a sinus infection when they are unable to drain out of the blocked sinuses. Frequent or persistent sinus infections may cause chronic sinus inflammation and symptoms. More than 50 percent of persons with moderate to severe asthma also have chronic sinusitis.

How is sinusitis treated?

If a bacterial infection is present, your doctor will carefully select an appropriate antibiotic to combat it. To reduce the inflammation, your doctor will also prescribe a corticosteroid nasal spray. When the inflammation decreases, the nasal passages will be less congested. Oral decongestants may also be helpful to reduce congestion. Topical decongestant nasal sprays are used with great caution since they can cause the vicious cycle of nasal stuffiness described earlier. Additional medications may be prescribed or obtained over the counter to help relieve the pain of sinusitis. Doctors also suggest nasal lavage with warm salt water or breathing in hot steam through the nose for 10 to 15 minutes, three to four times a day to make you feel more comfortable.

What's It Mean?

What are sinuses?

When people say, "I'm having a sinus attack," they usually are referring to symptoms of congestion and achiness in one or more of four pairs of cavities, or sinuses, known as *paranasal sinuses*. These cavities, located within the skull or bones of the head surrounding the nose, include the following:

- *Frontal sinuses* over the eyes in the brow area

- *Maxillary sinuses* inside each cheekbone

- *Ethmoid sinuses* just behind the bridge of the nose and between the eyes

- *Sphenoid sinuses* behind the ethmoids in the upper region of the nose and behind the eyes

Each sinus has an opening into the nose for the free exchange of air and mucus, and each is joined with the nasal passages by a continuous mucous membrane lining. Therefore, anything that causes a swelling in the nose—an infection, an allergic reaction, or another type of immune reaction—also can affect your sinuses.

Air trapped within a blocked sinus, along with pus or other secretions (liquid material) may cause pressure on the sinus wall. The result is the sometimes intense pain of a sinus attack. Similarly, when air is prevented from entering a paranasal sinus by a swollen membrane at the opening, a vacuum can be created that also causes pain.

Source: Excerpted from "Sinus Infection (Sinusitis)," National Institute of Allergy and Infectious Diseases (www3.niaid.nih.gov/topics/sinusitis/overview.htm), August 2007.

How can I prevent rhinitis and sinusitis?

The best course for preventing rhinitis and sinusitis is to keep your nasal passages as free and clear as possible. This is particularly important if you have allergies.

If you have chronic rhinitis and tend to get repeated bouts of sinusitis, your doctor may prescribe a steroid nasal spray. Taken every day, this medication will help to keep the nasal and sinus passages from becoming inflamed.

To the extent possible, avoid exposure to the things that trigger your allergies. Keep cigarette smoke out of your home and avoid it in other places as much as possible.

Most important, keep your doctor informed of your symptoms. Together you can devise a plan of action to take before a minor case of rhinitis or sinusitis turns into a bigger health problem.

♣ It's A Fact!!
Sinus Infection (Sinusitis) Overview

You're coughing, your nose is stuffy, and you feel tired and achy. You think that you might be getting a cold. Later, when the medicines you've been taking to relieve symptoms of the common cold are not working and you've got a terrible headache, you finally drag yourself to the doctor. After listening to your history of symptoms, examining your face and forehead, and perhaps doing a sinus x-ray, the doctor says you have sinusitis.

Sinusitis means your sinuses are infected or inflamed. But this gives little indication of the misery and pain this condition can cause. Health experts usually divide sinusitis cases into the following categories:

- Acute cases, which last for four weeks or less

- Subacute cases, which last four to 12 weeks

- Chronic cases, which last more than 12 weeks and can continue for months or even years

- Recurrent cases, which involve several acute attacks within a year

Health experts estimate 37 million Americans are affected by sinusitis every year. Health care providers report nearly 32 million cases of chronic sinusitis to the Centers for Disease Control and Prevention annually. Americans spend $5.8 billion each year on healthcare costs related to sinusitis.

Source: Excerpted from "Sinus Infection (Sinusitis)," National Institute of Allergy and Infectious Diseases (www3.niaid.nih.gov/topics/sinusitis/overview.htm), August 2007.

Part Five

Lifestyle Issues In Asthma Management

Chapter 39

Living With Asthma

Asthma is a long-term disease that requires long-term care. Successful asthma treatment requires you to take an active role in your care and follow your asthma action plan.

Learn How To Manage Your Asthma

Partner with your doctor to develop an asthma action plan. This plan will help you to properly take your medicines, identify your asthma triggers, and manage your disease if asthma symptoms worsen. Children age 10 or older— and younger children who can handle it—should be involved in developing and following their asthma action plan.

Most people who have asthma can successfully manage their symptoms at home by following their asthma action plans and having regular checkups. However, it's important to know when to seek emergency medical care.

Learn how to use your medicines correctly. If you take inhaled medicines, you should practice using your inhaler at your doctor's office. If you take long-term control medicines, take them daily as your doctor prescribes.

About This Chapter: Text in this chapter is from "Living with Asthma," National Heart, Lung and Blood Institute (www.nhlbi.nih.gov), September 2008.

Record your asthma symptoms as a way to track how well your asthma is controlled. Also, you may use a peak flow meter to measure and record how well your lungs are working.

Your doctor may ask you to keep records of your symptoms or peak flow results daily for a couple of weeks before an office visit and bring these records with you to the visit.

☞ Remember!!

- Asthma is a chronic (long-term) lung disease that inflames and narrows the airways and makes them more reactive to certain substances breathed in. The exact cause of asthma isn't known.

- Asthma affects people of all ages, but it most often starts in childhood. In the United States, more than 22 million people are known to have asthma. Nearly six million of these people are children.

- Asthma causes recurring periods of wheezing (a whistling sound when you breathe), chest tightness, shortness of breath, and coughing. The coughing often occurs at night or early in the morning.

- Sometimes symptoms are mild and go away on their own or after minimal treatment with an asthma medicine. Other times, the symptoms continue to get worse. When symptoms get more intense and/or additional symptoms appear, this is an asthma attack.

- It's important to treat asthma symptoms when you first notice them. This will help prevent the symptoms from worsening and causing a severe attack. Severe asthma attacks may require emergency care, and they can cause death.

- Your doctor will diagnose asthma based on your medical history, a physical exam, and results from tests. Asthma is difficult to diagnose in children younger than five years old.

- There's no cure for asthma. Asthma is a long-term disease that requires long-term care. Successful asthma treatment requires you to take an active role in your care. Learn how to manage your asthma, get ongoing care, and watch for signs that your asthma is getting worse.

These steps will help you keep track over time of how well you're controlling your asthma. This will help you spot problems early and prevent or relieve asthma attacks. Recording your symptoms and peak flow results to share with your doctor also will help him or her decide whether to adjust your treatment.

- The goal of asthma treatment is to control the disease by following the asthma action plan you create with your doctor, taking asthma medicines as prescribed, learning what things make your asthma worse and taking steps to avoid exposure to them, tracking your level of asthma control, and responding quickly to worsening symptoms.

- Asthma is treated with two types of medicines: long-term control medicines and quick-relief medicines. You use a device called an inhaler to take many of these medicines. This device allows the medicine to go right to your lungs.

- The amounts and types of medicine you need to treat your asthma depend on how well controlled your asthma is when you're closely following your asthma action plan. This may change over time.

- Call 911 for an ambulance to take you to the emergency room of your local hospital if you have trouble walking and talking because you're out of breath or you have blue lips or fingernails.

- Track your asthma by recording your symptoms, using a peak flow meter, and getting regular asthma checkups. Let your doctor know if your asthma is getting worse.

- Some aspects of treatment differ for people in certain age groups or those who have special needs.

- Most people who have asthma are able to manage the disease. They have few, if any, symptoms and can live normal, active lives.

Source: From "Key Points," National Heart, Lung and Blood Institute (www.nhlbi .nih.gov), September 2008.

Ongoing Care

Have regular asthma checkups with your doctor so he or she can assess your level of asthma control and adjust your treatment if needed. Remember, the main goal of asthma treatment is to achieve the best control of your asthma using the least amount of medicine. This may require frequent adjustments to your treatments.

If it's hard to follow your plan or the plan isn't working well, let your health care team know right away. They will work with you to adjust your plan to better suit your needs.

Get treatment for any other conditions that can interfere with your asthma management.

Watch For Signs That Your Asthma Is Getting Worse

Here are some signs that your asthma may be getting worse:

- Your symptoms start to occur more often, are more severe, and/or bother you at night and cause you to lose sleep.
- You're limiting your normal activities and missing school or work because of your asthma.
- Your peak flow number is low compared to your personal best or varies a lot from day to day.
- Your asthma medicines don't seem to work well anymore.
- You have to use your quick-relief inhaler more often. If you're using quick-relief medicine more than two days a week, your asthma isn't well controlled.
- You have to go to the emergency room or doctor because of an asthma attack.

If you have any of these signs, see your doctor. He or she may need to change your medicines or take other steps to control your asthma.

Partner with your health care team and take an active role in your care. This can help control asthma so it doesn't interfere with your activities and disrupt your life.

Chapter 40

Recognizing Asthma Symptoms And Triggers

What are the signs and symptoms of asthma?

Common asthma symptoms include the following:

- **Coughing:** Coughing from asthma is often worse at night or early in the morning, making it hard to sleep.

- **Wheezing:** Wheezing is a whistling or squeaky sound that occurs when you breathe.

- **Chest Tightness:** This may feel like something is squeezing or sitting on your chest.

- **Shortness Of Breath:** Some people who have asthma say they can't catch their breath or they feel out of breath. You may feel like you can't get air out of your lungs.

Not all people who have asthma have these symptoms. Likewise, having these symptoms doesn't always mean that you have asthma. A lung function test, done along with a medical history (including type and frequency of your symptoms) and physical exam, is the best way to diagnose asthma for certain.

About This Chapter: This chapter begins with "What Are the Signs and Symptoms of Asthma?" National Heart Lung and Blood Institute (www.nhlbi.nih.gov), September 2008. Additional information about emotional stress and asthma is cited separately within the chapter.

The types of asthma symptoms you have, how often they occur, and how severe they are may vary over time. Sometimes your symptoms may just annoy you. Other times they may be troublesome enough to limit your daily routine.

Severe symptoms can threaten your life. It's vital to treat symptoms when you first notice them so they don't become severe.

With proper treatment, most people who have asthma can expect to have few, if any, symptoms either during the day or at night.

What causes asthma symptoms to occur?

A number of things can bring about or worsen asthma symptoms. Your doctor will help you find out which things (sometimes called triggers) may cause your asthma to flare up if you come in contact with them. Triggers may include:

- allergens found in dust, animal fur, cockroaches, mold, and pollens from trees, grasses, and flowers;

- irritants such as cigarette smoke, air pollution, chemicals or dust in the workplace, compounds in home décor products, and sprays (such as hairspray);

- certain medicines such as aspirin or other nonsteroidal anti-inflammatory drugs and nonselective beta-blockers;

- sulfites in foods and drinks;

- viral upper respiratory infections such as colds;

- exercise (physical activity).

Other health conditions—such as runny nose, sinus infections, reflux disease, psychological stress, and sleep apnea—can make asthma more difficult to manage. These conditions need treatment as part of an overall asthma care plan.

Asthma is different for each person. Some of the factors listed may not affect you. Other factors that do affect you may not be on the list. Talk to your doctor about the things that seem to make your asthma worse.

Can Emotional Stress Exacerbate Asthma?

Originally published as "Can Emotional Stress Exacerbate Asthma?" written by Dr. Fred Little for The HealthCentral Network, Inc. and first published on HealthCentral's asthma website www.MyAsthmaCentral.com, March 16, 2007. Copyright © 2007 The HealthCentral Network, Inc. All Rights Reserved.

In this section, we discuss the connection between stress, stressful life events, and their effect on asthma control. While the connection is still being worked out, there is evidence not only from clinical experience, but in research studies in humans and animals that stress can aggravate asthma.

Stress And Asthma

There are many stressors that worsen asthma control in patients with asthma. These include allergens (such as cat dander and pollen), irritants (e.g., smoke), and cold infections. These are usually considered 'exposures', and we try to identify these triggers and avoid them if we can. Similarly, stress can be thought of as a type of exposure, though a psychological one, which can trigger asthma. Many patients find that stressful situations make them feel short of breath and wheeze, and that they need to use their quick relief inhaler for relief.

Stressful life events, which are less immediate, can also lead to worsened asthma control in certain individuals. A recent study measured quality of life related to asthma in a range of individuals and found that in people with similar *baseline* asthma severity, asthma control was poorer in subsets of individuals who had recent stressful life events, such as divorce or moving. Another study, in children, found that the beneficial response to sublingual immunotherapy (similar to allergy shots) was decreased in children with stressful lives and life events. While the mechanism by which stress and stressful life events worsens asthma control, it is clear from the clinic and research studies that the connection is clear.

What About Stress And Asthma In Animal Models

To better understand this connection, researchers have tried to replicate what is known in humans using animal models. In an animal model of asthma in mice, studies have shown that stressing animals leads to changes in the asthmatic response. These changes were found at different stages of developing asthma in these models, both early and late. Researchers hope that these models of stress and asthma will improve our understanding of the way that stress causes worsening asthma control.

Closing Thoughts

Clearly, avoiding stress is not as easy an 'exposure' to avoid as other asthma triggers, such as pets and pollens. But being aware of this direct connection is important for all patients with asthma. Your doctor can help you to better control your asthma, especially for triggers that are less typical and like stress, poorly understood.

♣ It's A Fact!!
Can asthma be prevented?

Currently, there isn't a way to prevent asthma from starting in the first place. However, you can take steps to control the disease and prevent its symptoms.

- Learn about your asthma and how to control it.

- Follow your written asthma action plan. (See the National Heart, Lung, and Blood Institute's Asthma Action Plan as a sample; available online at http://www.nhlbi.nih.gov/health/public/lung/asthma/asthma_actplan.htm.)

- Use medicines as your doctor directs.

- Identify and avoid things that make your asthma worse (as much as you can).

- Keep track of your asthma symptoms and level of control.

- Get regular checkups for your asthma.

Source: National Heart Lung and Blood Institute (www.nhlbi.nih.gov), September 2008.

Chapter 41

Air Pollution And Outdoor Triggers

When you're outdoors, you have less control over the triggers you encounter. You can't, for example, vacuum the lawn if pollen is bothering you, and there's no air cleaner large enough to clean a city's air pollution.

Still, there are things you can do to help reduce your exposure to outdoor triggers. By making a few adjustments, and by taking your medication as directed, you can breathe easier when you're outside.

Molds

Molds are asthma triggers for many people. A type of fungus, their spores float in the air where they're easily inhaled and can lead to coughing, sneezing, wheezing, and chest tightness.

You'll find molds wherever it's damp. This includes piles of vegetation, stagnant water, and garbage containers.

About This Chapter: This chapter begins with "Air Pollution and Outdoor Triggers," reprinted with permission from the Asthma Society of Canada, © 2009. All rights reserved. For additional information about asthma, visit http://www.asthma.ca. Additional text under the heading "Outdoor Air Pollution," is from the U.S. Environmental Protection Agency, 2009.

Pollens

Pollens are a very common trigger for asthma symptoms. Generated by trees, grasses and weeds, airborne pollens are easily inhaled, especially during warm-weather months.

If you're allergic to pollen, there are a number of things you can do to stay healthy:

- Use a HEPA-filtered air cleaner.

- Plant low-allergen gardens.

- On days when the pollen count is high, use an air conditioner in your home and car, and also try to keep your windows closed as much as possible.

> ✔ **Quick Tip**
>
> If you're sensitive to mold spores, try the following:
>
> • have piles of grass removed from your lawn immediately after it's mowed;
>
> • when leaves accumulate on your lawn, have them raked and re-moved;
>
> • keep garbage cans clean;
>
> • have outdoor containers that hold stagnant water removed;
>
> • ensure that gutters on your house face away from the house.
>
> Source: © 2009 Asthma Society of Canada.

- If you usually exercise outdoors, con-sider exercising inside on days when the pollen count is high.

- Avoid going outside between 5 and 10 a.m. on hot and windy days.

- Check the pollen count to see whether you should reduce the amount of time you spend outdoors.

- Shower and change your clothing if you've been outdoors on a high-pollen-count day.

- If there are plants in your yard that trigger symptoms, have someone remove them.

- Use a good furnace filter and change it regularly.

- Do not place trees or plants near windows, or near the air-intake of your furnace or air conditioner.

- Do not hang your laundry out to dry—use a clothes dryer instead.

- Do not touch plants that you think might be triggers—and if you do, wash your hands immediately afterwards.

Cold Air

Cold air, or sudden changes in the weather, can also trigger asthma symptoms. If you're affected by the cold, the following tips can help:

- Try breathing through your nose. This helps warm the air before it reaches your lungs.

- If you have to breathe through your mouth, wear a scarf or a special cold-weather mask to help humidify and warm the air you breathe, making it easier on your lungs.

- Exercise indoors on cold days.

Air Pollutants

While air pollution as a cause of asthma has not been verified, there is good evidence that pollution causes the symptoms of many people with asthma to get worse on days when the air-quality index is high.

If you find your symptoms become worse on these days, try to:

- reduce the amount of time you spend outside when air-pollution is high;

- exercise indoors if you usually exercise outdoors;

- turn on the air conditioner in your home and car and keep your windows closed.

Outdoor Air Pollution

Small particles and ozone come from things like exhaust from cars and factories, smoke, and road dust. When inhaled, outdoor pollutants can aggravate the lungs, and can lead to chest pain, coughing, shortness of breath, and throat irritation. Outdoor air pollution may also worsen chronic respiratory diseases, such as asthma. On days when ozone air pollution is highest, ozone has been associated with 10–20 percent of all respiratory hospital visits and admissions.

Watch for the Air Quality Index, or AQI, during your local weather report. The AQI is a tool that offers you clear information every day on whether air quality in your area could be a health risk. The AQI uses colors to show how much pollution is in the air. Green and yellow mean air pollution levels are low. Orange, red, or purple mean pollution is at levels that may make asthma worse.

Actions You Can Take

State agencies will use television and radio to notify citizens of ozone alerts. On days when your state or local air pollution control agency calls an Ozone Action Day, people with asthma should limit prolonged physical activity outdoors. Consider adjusting outdoor activities to early in the morning or later in the evening.

✔ Quick Tip

On Ozone Action Days, you can do the following 10 things to help keep ozone formation to a minimum:

- Instead of driving, share a ride, walk, or bike.

- Take public transportation.

- If you must drive, avoid excessive idling and jackrabbit starts.

- Don't refuel your car or only do so after 7 p.m.

- Avoid using outboard motors, off-road vehicles, or other gasoline powered recreational vehicles.

- Defer mowing your lawn until late evening or the next day. Also avoid using gasoline-powered garden equipment.

- Postpone chores that use oil-based paints, solvents, or varnishes that produce fumes.

- If you are barbecuing, use an electric starter instead of charcoal lighter fluid.

- Limit or postpone household chores that will involve the use of consumer products.

- Conserve energy in your home to reduce energy needs.

Source: "Outdoor Air Pollution," U.S. Environmental Protection Agency, 2009.

Chapter 42

Controlling Asthma Triggers In The Home

Indoor Triggers—Home And Work

With smog, pollen and severe weather changes, you might think that you're more likely to encounter more triggers outdoors than indoors. In fact, the opposite is true. Canadians spend 90 percent of their time indoors. This, along with changes in how our homes are built, has lead to poor indoor air quality and more triggers, in our homes.

Fortunately, a great deal has been learned about asthma triggers that exist inside. By educating yourself about indoor hazards, you'll discover simple ways to reduce their levels.

Dust Mites: Dust mite allergy is a common problem for people with asthma. The excretions and body parts of these tiny, spider-like creatures can be a powerful trigger of asthma symptoms.

Dust mites congregate in soft-surfaced places where there is an abundant food supply. Dust mites feed off shed human skin and are thus found in bedding, mattresses, pillows, sofas and carpets.

Effective strategies for minimizing dust mites are:

About This Chapter: This chapter begins with information from "Indoor Triggers—Home & Work," reprinted with permission from the Asthma Society of Canada, © 2009. All rights reserved. For additional information about asthma, visit http://www.asthma.ca.

✔ Quick Tip

10 Steps To Making Your Home Asthma Friendly

1. Take it outside. One of the most common asthma triggers in the home is second-hand smoke. Until you can quit, smoke outside, not in your home or car.

2. Good night, little mite! Dust mites are also triggers for asthma. For mite population control, cover mattresses and pillows with dust-proof (allergen impermeable) zippered covers. Wash sheets and blankets once a week in hot water.

3. Play it Safe. Ozone and particle pollution can cause asthma attacks. Watch for the Air Quality index (AQI) during your local weather report. When AQI reports unhealthy levels, limit outdoor activities.

4. A little goes a long way. Reduce everyday dust build-up, by regularly dusting with a damp cloth and vacuuming carpet and fabric-covered furniture.

5. Stake your claim. Household pets can trigger asthma with skin flakes, urine, and saliva. Keep pets outdoors, if possible.

6. Uninvite unwelcome guests. Cockroaches can trigger asthma. Don't invite them into your home by leaving food or garbage out. Always clean up messes and spills and store food in airtight containers.

7. Think before you spray. Instead of pesticide sprays, control pests by using baits or traps. If sprays are necessary, always circulate fresh air into the room being treated and keep asthma sufferers out of that room for several hours after any spraying.

8. Break the mold. Mold is another asthma trigger. The key to controlling mold is controlling moisture. Wash and dry hard surfaces to prevent and remove mold. Replace moldy ceiling tiles and carpet.

9. Air it out. Reducing the moisture will control asthma triggers like mold, cockroaches, and dust mites. Use exhaust fans or open windows when cooking and showering. Fix leaky plumbing or other unwanted sources of water.

10. Plan before the attack. Work with your doctor or health care provider to develop a written asthma management plan that includes information on your triggers and how to manage them.

Post a note. Post this plan on your refrigerator to help control asthma triggers and reduce asthma attacks in your home.

Source: "Clearing the Air of Asthma Triggers: 10 Steps to Making Your Home Asthma-Friendly," U.S. Environmental Protection Agency (www.epa.gov), May 2004.

- use a dehumidifier in damp area. Keep the humidity level below 50 percent. Dust mites can't survive in dry environments.

- remove carpets, especially in the bedroom;

- launder bed linens in very hot water (131 degrees Fahrenheit).

- Encase your pillow, mattress and box spring in mite-allergen impermeable encasings.

Cockroaches: Cockroaches are one of most hated household pests, and for good reason. Not only are they a terrible nuisance, their feces have been shown to trigger symptoms in individuals with asthma.

If your home has cockroaches, make sure that food and water are never left where they can get at them. To ensure they leave and never come back, call a professional exterminator.

Indoor Molds: Molds are fungus that can be found just about anywhere it's damp and where air flow is minimal, like basements and bathrooms. Their airborne spores can trigger asthma symptoms, but there are many ways to avoid them. The best way is to keep your home dry and clean.

- Monitor the humidity level in your home with a hygrometer and keep the level between 40–45 percent.

- Make sure your home is well ventilated.

- Remove carpeting where possible. If carpet is kept, vacuum thoroughly and frequently using a vacuum cleaner with a high efficiency particulate air (HEPA) filter.

- Clean moldy areas, especially in bathrooms, with an anti-mold cleaner like vinegar or a chlorine-bleach solution. When using these chemicals, be sure to use them in a well-ventilated area.

- Ensure that you have proper drainage around your house.

- Use a dehumidifier if humidity is higher than 50 percent (basements).

- Always use bathroom and kitchen fans.

- Reduce your number of house plants.

- Do not have carpet in bathrooms or directly on concrete floors in the basement.

Chemical Fumes: Many people with asthma are affected by airborne chemicals. They may be exposed to them in the home, or even at work.

At home, chemicals are reasonably easy to control. If you have paints or other volatile products in your house, you can get rid of them or seal them

✔ Quick Tip

To determine whether you've developed occupational asthma, ask yourself the following questions:

- Did your asthma symptoms appear within weeks or months of starting a new job, or moving to a new area within your current job?

- Do your asthma symptoms regularly and predictably occur while you're at work or within a few hours of leaving the workplace?

- Do you notice that your symptoms improve on weekends or when you're on vacation, and then get worse when you go back to work?

- Do other people at work have the same symptoms?

If you suspect you have occupational asthma, talk to your doctor, who may refer you to a pulmonologist for further assessment.

If your employer has taken every preventive measure possible and your symptoms are still severe, you may have to consider switching careers. Remember, you can always talk to your doctor if you think your job is making you sick.

Source: © 2009 Asthma Society of Canada.

carefully and place them in a garage or shed. If you're sensitive to heavy perfumes, try not to use products that use them.

Occupational Asthma: If you have any of the following jobs, you may be at risk for occupational asthma:

- Grains, flours, plants and gums: Bakers, chemists, and farmers

- Animals, insects and fungi: Poultry workers, entomologists, laboratory workers, and veterinary professionals

- Chemicals: Aircraft fitters, brewery workers, pulp mill workers, electronic workers, hairdressers, refrigeration workers, resin manufacturers and dye weighers

- Isocyanates and metals: Car sprayers, boat builders, foam, TDI [toluene diisocyanate] and refrigerator manufacturers, platinum chemists and refiners, printers and laminators and welders

- Drugs and enzymes: Ampicillin, detergent and enzyme manufacturers, pharmacists and pharmaceutical workers

- Woods: Carpenters, millers, saw-mill workers, wood finishers and machinists

Chapter 43

What People With Asthma Should Know About Pets

Who gets pet allergies?

Six out of 10 people in the United States come in contact with cats or dogs. The total pet population is more than 100 million, or about four pets for every 10 people.

Allergies to pets with fur or feathers are common, especially among people who have other allergies or asthma. From 15 percent to 30 percent of people with allergies have allergic reactions to cats and dogs.

People with dog allergies may be allergic to all dogs or to only some breeds. Cat allergies are about twice as common as dog allergies.

What causes a pet allergy?

The job of immune system cells is to find foreign substances such as viruses and bacteria and get rid of them. Normally, this response protects us from dangerous diseases. People with pet allergies have supersensitive immune systems

About This Chapter: This chapter begins with information from "Pet Allergies," © 2005 Asthma and Allergy Foundation of America (www.aafa.org). All rights reserved. Reprinted with permission. Additional information about exposure to pets and its impact on kids is cited separately in the chapter.

that react to harmless proteins in the pet's dander (dead skin that is shed), saliva, or urine. These proteins are called allergens.

Dogs and cats secrete fluids and shed dander that contain the allergens. They collect on fur and other surfaces. The allergens will not lose their strength for a long time, sometimes for several months. They appear to be sticky and adhere to walls, clothing and other surfaces.

What are the symptoms?

Reactions to cat and dog allergens that land on the membranes that line eyes and nose include swelling and itching of the membranes, stuffy nose, and inflamed eyes. A pet scratch or lick can cause the skin area to become red.

If allergen levels are low or sensitivity is minor, symptoms may not appear until after several days of contact with the pet.

♣ It's A Fact!!

Pet hair is not an allergen. It can collect dander, though. It also harbors other allergens like dust and pollen.

Cat and dog allergens are everywhere. Pet dander is even in homes never occupied by these animals because it is carried on people's clothing. The allergens get in the air with petting, grooming, or stirring the air where the allergens have settled. Once airborne, the particles can stay suspended in the air for long periods of time.

Source: © 2005 Asthma and Allergy Foundation of America.

Many airborne particles are small enough to get into the lungs. When inhaled, the allergens combine with antibodies. This can cause severe breathing problems—coughing, wheezing and shortness of breath—in highly sensitive people within 15 to 30 minutes. Sometimes highly sensitive people also get an intense rash on the face, neck and upper chest.

For about 20 percent to 30 percent of people with asthma, cat contact can trigger a severe asthma attack. Cat allergies also can lead to chronic asthma.

How is a pet allergy diagnosed?

If a pet allergy is suspected, the doctor may diagnose it by taking a medical history and testing the blood of the patient. Some people are so attached to their pets that they will deny the pets could cause their symptoms. In these cases, the patient is removed from the animal's environment to see if symptoms go away. It does not help to remove the dog or cat. Allergens still in the area can cause symptoms months after the animal is gone.

To diagnose cat-induced asthma, the patient must have both of the following:

- Asthma symptoms when exposed to cat or cat allergen

- An allergic reaction to a skin test or to a blood test called RAST (radioallergosorbent test). To make sure the diagnosis is correct, the doctor will watch what happens when a cat is added then removed from the patient's environment several times.

What is the best treatment?

The best treatment is to avoid contact with cats or dogs or their dander. Keep the pets out of the house, and avoid visiting people with pets. Avoiding cats and dogs may give you enough relief that you will not need medication.

Keeping the pet outdoors will help, but will not rid the house of pet allergens. Another option is to have pets that do not have fur or feathers. Fish, snakes or turtles are some choices.

Asthma And Pets: Is Exposure To Pets Harmful Or Beneficial To Kids?

From "Asthma and Pets: Is Exposure to Pets Harmful or Beneficial to Kids?" reprinted with permission from www.LungDiseaseFocus.com. © Morefocus Media, Inc.

According to the National Heart, Lung and Blood Institute, the number of asthma and allergy cases is on the rise: nearly twice as many cases are currently reported as compared to twenty years ago. What has caused this drastic increase?

Scientists are working frantically to figure out what can be done to reverse this trend. While no conclusive solution has emerged yet, some interesting theories are being tested. One of the leading theories, known as the hygiene hypothesis, examines the potential risks of "over-cleanliness" versus

☞ Remember!!
What if I want to keep my pet?

To test the effect of household pets on your quality of life, remove them from your home for at least two months and clean thoroughly every week. After two months, if you still want pets, bring a pet into the house. Measure the change in your symptoms, then decide if the change in your symptoms is worth keeping the pet.

If you decide to keep a pet, bar it from the bedroom. You spend from one-third to one-half of your time there. Keep the bedroom door closed and clean the bedroom aggressively:

- Because animal allergens are sticky, you must remove the animal's favorite furniture, remove wall-to-wall carpet and scrub the walls and woodwork. Keep surfaces throughout the home clean and uncluttered. Bare floors and walls are best.

- If you must have carpet, select ones with a low pile and steam clean them frequently. Better yet, use throw rugs that can be washed in hot water.

- Wear a dust mask to vacuum. Vacuum cleaners stir up allergens that have settled on carpet and make allergies worse. Use a vacuum with a HEPA (high efficiency particulate air) filter if possible.

- Forced-air heating and air-conditioning can spread allergens through the house. Cover bedroom vents with dense filtering material like cheesecloth.

- Adding an air cleaner with a HEPA filter to central heating and air conditioning can help remove pet allergens from the air. The air cleaner should be used at least four hours per day. Another type of air cleaner that has an electrostatic filter will remove particles the size of animal allergens from the air. No air cleaner or filter will remove allergens stuck to surfaces, though.

- Washing the pet every week may reduce airborne allergens, but is of questionable value in reducing a person's symptoms.

- Have someone without a pet allergy brush the pet outside to remove dander as well as clean the litter box or cage.

Source: © 2005 Asthma and Allergy Foundation of America.

the potential benefits of allergen exposure at a young age. However, the hygiene hypothesis is still highly controversial.

The Hygiene Hypothesis: Modern, sterile living conditions result in less exposure to a variety of toxins and microorganisms at an early age. The hygiene hypothesis suggests that this reduced contact with potential allergens has ironically caused the surge in allergy and asthma cases.

Simply, the argument claims that a lack of exposure to these stimuli is detrimental to the developing immune system, placing individuals at a greater risk of overreacting when they are eventually exposed to allergic triggers later in life. Essentially, the hygiene hypothesis asserts that the immune system should be tested and trained at a young age in order to be properly balanced.

Mixed Results: Compelling scientific evidence supports the hygiene hypothesis. Several studies have been published providing support for the notion that kids who grow up in homes with cats and dogs have far fewer problems with allergies and asthma. The research argues that exposure to animal dander and the rich variety of allergens associated with pets stimulates the production of the immune system's T-cells early on.

However, in the last couple of years there has been a backlash in the scientific community: recent reports claim that exposure to dogs and cats at a young age can actually increase the risk of developing asthma and allergies. Clearly, the validity of the hygiene hypothesis is still in question.

The Complicated Truth About Asthma: What can we make of all of this, and what is the consensus of the research results? Unfortunately, it remains unclear whether having pets at home bears any weight at all on preventing or promoting the development of asthma and allergies. What does remain clear, however, is that people who have already developed asthma or allergies should avoid potential triggers such as animal dander, pollen, and tobacco smoke.

An Answer In Sight: Part of the difficulty in obtaining conclusive evidence in this debate is the complexity of designing a properly controlled study. Because cat and dog allergens are present everywhere, non-pet owners have often already been exposed.

A three-and-a-half-year research study, which began in 2001, was designed to reveal how exposure to cat, dog, and mite allergens in developing children would affect their development of asthma and allergies later in life. This ongoing study, under the direction of members of the North West Lung Research Centre in Manchester, UK, differs from others in that it is performed longitudinally over a long period of time and is stringently controlled.

Two groups are under observation: an active group with strict instructions and hygienic guidelines intended to reduce the level of allergens in the home and a control group. Hopefully, the results of this study will provide a better idea of whether having pets at home influences our health.

Chapter 44

Using An Asthma Action Plan

How Is Asthma Treated And Controlled?

Asthma is a long-term disease that can't be cured. The goal of asthma treatment is to control the disease. Good asthma control will accomplish the following goals:

- Prevent chronic and troublesome symptoms such as coughing and shortness of breath

- Reduce the need for quick-relief medicines

- Help maintain good lung function

- Help maintain normal activity levels and sleep through the night

- Prevent asthma attacks that could result in trips to the emergency room or being admitted to the hospital for treatment

To reach these goals, you should actively partner with your doctor to manage your asthma. Children age 10 or older—and younger children who are able—should take an active role in their asthma care.

About This Chapter: Text in this chapter begins with text excerpted from "How is Asthma Treated and Controlled?" National Heart Lung and Blood Institute (NHLBI), September 2008. Text under the headings "Asthma Action Plan," and "How To Control Things That Make Your Asthma Worse," is from "Asthma Action Plan," NHLBI, 2007.

☞ **Remember!!**

Taking an active role to control asthma involves working with your doctor and other clinicians on your health care team to create and follow an *asthma action plan*. It also means avoiding factors that can make your asthma flare up and treating other conditions that can interfere with asthma management.

Source: NHLBI, September 2008.

An asthma action plan gives guidance on taking medicines properly, avoiding factors that worsen asthma, tracking the level of asthma control, responding to worsening asthma, and seeking emergency care when needed.

Asthma is treated with two types of medicines: long-term control and quick-relief medicines. Long-term control medicines help reduce airway inflammation and prevent asthma symptoms. Quick-relief, or "rescue," medicines relieve asthma symptoms that may flare up.

Your initial asthma treatment will depend on how severe your disease is. Follow-up asthma treatment will depend on how well your asthma action plan is working to control your symptoms and prevent you from having asthma attacks.

Your level of asthma control can vary over time and with changes in your home, school, or work environments that alter how often you are exposed to the factors that can make your asthma worse. Your doctor may need to increase your medicine if your asthma doesn't stay under control.

On the other hand, if your asthma is well controlled for several months, your doctor may be able to decrease your medicine. These adjustments either up or down to your medicine will help you maintain the best control possible with the least amount of medicine necessary.

Asthma treatment for certain groups of people, such as children, pregnant women, or those for whom exercise brings on asthma symptoms, will need to be adjusted to meet their special needs.

Follow An Asthma Action Plan

Work with your doctor to create a personal written asthma action plan. The asthma action plan shows your daily treatment, such as what kind of medicines to take and when to take them. The plan explains when to call the doctor or go to the emergency room.

If a child has asthma, all of the people who care for him or her should know about the child's asthma action plan. This includes babysitters and workers at daycare centers, schools, and camps. These caretakers can help the child follow his or her action plan.

Details about what is included in an asthma plan can be found in the asthma action plan described in this chapter, beginning on the next page.

Avoid Things That Can Worsen Your Asthma

A number of common things (sometimes called *asthma triggers*) can set off or worsen asthma symptoms. Once you know what these factors are, you can take steps to control many of them.

For example, if exposure to pollens or air pollution makes your asthma worse, try to limit time outdoors when the levels of these substances are high in the outdoor air. If animal fur sets off your asthma symptoms, keep pets with fur out of your home or bedroom. The National Heart Lung and Blood Institute (NHLBI) offers many useful tips for controlling things that make your asthma worse.

If your asthma symptoms are clearly linked to allergies, and you can't avoid exposure to those allergens, then your doctor may advise you to get allergy shots for the specific allergens that bother your asthma. You may need to see a specialist if you're thinking about getting allergy shots. These shots may lessen or prevent your asthma symptoms, but they can't cure your asthma.

Several health conditions can make asthma more difficult to manage. These conditions include runny nose, sinus infections, reflux disease, psychological stress, and sleep apnea. Your doctor will treat these conditions as well.

Asthma Action Plan

For: _____ Date: _____

Doctor: _____ Doctor's Phone Number: _____

Hospital/Emergency Department Phone Number: _____

Green Zone: Doing Well

- No cough, wheeze, chest tightness, or shortness of breath during the day or night

- Can do usual activities

And, if a peak flow meter is used:

Peak flow: more than _____
(80 percent or more of my best peak flow)

My best peak flow is: _____

Take these long-term control medicines each day
(include an anti-inflammatory):

Medicine	How much to take	When to take it
_____	_____	_____
_____	_____	_____
_____	_____	_____
_____	_____	_____

Take these medicines before exercise if your asthma is exercise-induced.

Medicine	How much to take *2 or 4 puffs*	When to take it *5 to 60 minutes before*
_____	_____	_____
_____	_____	_____
_____	_____	_____
_____	_____	_____

Yellow Zone: Asthma Is Getting Worse

- Cough, wheeze, chest tightness, or shortness of breath, or

- Waking at night due to asthma, or

- Can do some, but not all, usual activities

Or:

Peak flow: _____ to _____
(50 to 79 percent of my best peak flow)

First: Add quick-relief medicine—and keep taking your GREEN ZONE medicine.

Take short-acting beta$_2$-agonist _____

- __ 2 or __ 4 puffs, every 20 minutes for up to 1 hour

- __ Nebulizer, once

Second: If your symptoms (and peak flow, if used) return to GREEN ZONE after 1 hour of above treatment:

Continue monitoring to be sure you stay in the green zone.

Or:

If your symptoms (and peak flow, if used) do not return to GREEN ZONE after 1 hour of above treatment:

Take short-acting beta$_2$-agonist _____

- __ 2 or __ 4 puffs, every 20 minutes for up to 1 hour

- __ Nebulizer, once

Add oral steroid: _____

- _____ mg per day

- For _____ (3–10) days

- Call the doctor __ before / within _____ hours after taking the oral steroid.

Red Zone: Medical Alert!

- Very short of breath, or

- Quick-relief medicines have not helped, or

- Cannot do usual activities, or

- Symptoms are same or get worse after 24 hours in Yellow Zone

Or:

Peak flow: less than _____
(50 percent of my best peak flow)

Take this medicine:

Short-acting beta$_2$-agonist _____

____ 4 puffs, ___ 6 puffs or, ___ Nebulizer

Oral steroid _____ mg

Then call your doctor NOW.

Go to the hospital or call an ambulance if:

- You are still in the red zone after 15 minutes AND

- You have not reached your doctor.

Danger Signs

- Trouble walking and talking due to shortness of breath

- Lips or fingernails are blue

- Take 4 or 6 puffs of your quick-relief medicine AND

- Go to the hospital or call for an ambulance at
(phone) _____ NOW!

How To Control Things That Make Your Asthma Worse

The following list suggests things you can do to avoid your asthma triggers. Learn what triggers make your asthma worse and ask your doctor to help you find out if you have other triggers as well. Then decide with your doctor what steps you will take.

Allergens

Animal Dander: Some people are allergic to the flakes of skin or dried saliva from animals with fur or feathers. The best thing to do in this situation is to keep furred or feathered pets out of your home. If you can't keep the pet outdoors, then keep the pet out of your bedroom and other sleeping areas at all times, and keep the door closed. Also, remove carpets and furniture covered with cloth from your home. If that is not possible, keep the pet away from fabric-covered furniture and carpets.

Dust Mites: Many people with asthma are allergic to dust mites. Dust mites are tiny bugs that are found in every home—in mattresses, pillows, carpets, upholstered furniture, bedcovers, clothes, stuffed toys, and fabric or other fabric-covered items.

If you are allergic to dust mites encase your mattress in a special dust-proof cover. Encase your pillow in a special dust-proof cover or wash the pillow each week in hot water. Water must be hotter than 130° F to kill the mites. Cold or warm water used with detergent and bleach can also be effective. Wash the sheets and blankets on your bed each week in hot water. Try not to sleep or lie on cloth-covered cushions. Remove carpets from your bedroom and those laid on concrete, if you can. Keep stuffed toys out of the bed or wash the toys weekly in hot water or cooler water with detergent and bleach.

Reduce indoor humidity to below 60 percent (ideally between 30–50 percent). Dehumidifiers or central air conditioners can do this.

Cockroaches: Many people with asthma are allergic to the dried droppings and remains of cockroaches. Keep food and garbage in closed containers. Never leave food out. Use poison baits, powders, gels, or paste (for example, boric acid). You can also use traps. If a spray is used to kill roaches, stay out of the room until the odor goes away.

Indoor Mold: To prevent indoor mold, fix leaky faucets, pipes, or other sources of water that have mold around them, and clean moldy surfaces with a cleaner that has bleach in it.

Pollen And Outdoor Mold: During your allergy season, when pollen or mold spore counts are high, these steps can help you avoid symptom triggers: Try to keep your windows closed. Stay indoors with windows closed from late morning to afternoon, if you can. Pollen and some mold spore counts are highest at that time. Ask your doctor whether you need to take or increase anti-inflammatory medicine before your allergy season starts

Irritants

Tobacco Smoke: If you smoke, ask your doctor for ways to help you quit. Ask family members to quit smoking, too. Do not allow smoking in your home or car

Smoke, Strong Odors, And Sprays: If possible, do not use a wood-burning stove, kerosene heater, or fireplace. Try to stay away from strong odors and sprays, such as perfume, talcum powder, hair spray, and paints.

Vacuum Cleaning: Try to get someone else to vacuum for you once or twice a week, if you can. Stay out of rooms while they are being vacuumed and for a short while afterward. If you vacuum, use a dust mask (from a hardware store), a double-layered or microfilter vacuum cleaner bag, or a vacuum cleaner with a HEPA filter.

✔ Quick Tip Managing Other Things That Can Make Asthma Worse

Sulfites In Foods And Beverages: Teens should not drink alcoholic beverages, but you should know that beer and wine can cause asthma symptoms. Do not eat dried fruit, processed potatoes, or shrimp if they cause asthma symptoms.

Cold Air: Cover your nose and mouth with a scarf on cold or windy days.

Other Medicines: Tell your doctor about all the medicines you take. Include cold medicines, aspirin, vitamins and other supplements, and nonselective beta-blockers (including those in eye drops).

Source: NHLBI, 2007.

Chapter 45

Calming Your Cough

Cough, cough, cough. That maddening cough that never goes away. The cough that makes people in the grocery store cover their carts as they speed past you. The cough that hammers a classroom of students trying to take a test or learn a new concept. Why do we cough? What can we do about it?

Minnesota allergist Pramod Kelkar, MD, chair of the American Academy of Allergy, Asthma and Immunology Cough Committee, answers our cough questions.

What are the different causes of coughs?

Dr. Kelkar: Coughing is a reflex and usually happens involuntarily; it's your body's natural reaction to an irritated airway. Often, it is a symptom of an underlying disease. For instance, chronic "it-won't-go-away" coughing can indicate that asthma, allergies, or GERD (gastroesophageal reflux disease) is out of control.

Coughing is also the body's way of clearing mucus in the airways or getting rid of foreign materials such as allergens, irritating pollutants or secondhand smoke that enter the respiratory tract (the nose, throat, larynx, sinuses, or lungs).

Physicians divide coughs into three categories:

1. Acute cough is a cough that lasts less than two to three weeks. Most often it is caused by the common cold or other upper respiratory tract viral infections, bronchitis, pneumonia, allergies, asthma, or sinusitis.

2. Subacute cough is a cough that lasts from three to eight weeks. It is often caused by the same diseases that cause acute cough but becomes more serious if not treated.

3. Chronic cough is a cough that lasts longer than eight weeks (or four weeks in children). The three most common causes of chronic cough are postnasal drip/drainage, asthma, and GERD.

Can you tell what's causing a cough by how it sounds or feels?

Dr. Kelkar: Not really. Figuring out the exact cause of cough can be challenging. Whooping cough will obviously have whooping sound in most cases (but not always). Barking or honking cough in children can sometimes be from habit (again, not always). In adults, the types of cough do not give a specific indication about a specific diagnosis.

That's why it's important to consider all symptoms. For example, allergies are associated with nose and sinus problems; asthma can produce chest tightness, wheezing and shortness of breath; and GERD often causes heartburn and a sour taste in the mouth. Having said that, it is important to keep in mind that all these diseases can occur with cough as the only symptom and multiple conditions can occur in the same patient (such as asthma and GERD).

When should patients see a doctor about a cough?

Dr. Kelkar: Cough in children less than six months old must always be evaluated. In other children, any wet cough or coughing while feeding should be checked by a physician.

Many cold- and virus-related coughs go away within a couple of weeks. If a cough lasts more than two weeks, however, you should see your healthcare provider.

Remember!!

For patients of all ages, seek medical help as soon as possible if you experience any of the following:

- Coughing up blood or yellow-green sputum/ phlegm

- A temperature higher than 101 degrees F

- Losing weight

- Night sweats

- Feeling short of breath and tight in the chest

- No relief from over-the-counter medications or other medicines

- Coughing all night long

- Coughing that changes in character or becomes worse/deeper

- Coughing accompanied by a high-pitched sound or stridor while inhaling

What type of physician should patients see for a cough?

Dr. Kelkar: Common types of acute and subacute cough can be treated initially by any healthcare professional. If the cough lasts more than four weeks, however, your physician may suggest you consult a specialist, such as an allergist. Trained to treat upper and lower respiratory disorders, allergists can be an important part of your healthcare team, guiding patients to specific testing, referrals, and a comprehensive treatment plan.

What should you expect at your visit with a healthcare provider?

Dr. Kelkar: First of all, your provider will gather information from you, like how long you've had the cough, how it started, what triggers it, accompanying symptoms, when the cough occurs, whether there is fever, and whether there is any phlegm/ sputum and what color it is. This will be followed by a detailed physical examination to detect signs of any underlying disease such as swelling in your nose, drainage on the back of your throat from allergies, or wheezing from asthma.

Some patients may require an x-ray or specialized tests based on the suspected cause of the cough: skin prick tests for allergies, breathing tests and spirometry for asthma, or imaging study (CAT scans) for sinuses. Your healthcare provider may refer you to an appropriate specialist like an allergist or pulmonologist for some of these tests.

What medications might a physician prescribe for coughing?

Dr. Kelkar: Your physician will diagnose and treat the cause of your cough, not just the cough itself. Sometimes, your physician will recommend trying a particular medication to see if it's effective before doing expensive and invasive testing.

For instance, allergies can be treated by oral antihistamines, corticosteroid nose sprays, and allergy shots. Asthma can be treated with bronchodilator inhalers and inhaled corticosteroids and by avoiding allergens and irritants that cause symptoms. (Asthma patients who need daily medications for their breathing symptoms should see an allergist to identify specific allergies.) GERD requires medications as well as a change in diet and lifestyle such as avoiding caffeinated beverages, alcohol, acidic fruit juices, chocolate, smoking, and not lying down immediately after a meal.

Are there issues with chronic cough that are specific to children?

Dr. Kelkar: Coughing in children may occur from a variety of causes, some of which are specific to children, including croup, bronchiolitis, RSV infection, a tic-disorder manifesting as a dry cough, and exposure to cigarette smoke from parents/caregivers. Sometimes a foreign body such as a toy or a food item will get stuck in a child's airway and cause a cough that goes on for days or weeks before it is detected.

Because young children cannot communicate in detail, it is challenging to treat coughs at home without a physician's guidance. Parents and caregivers should talk with their healthcare team before using over-the-counter medications in children and not give more than the label recommends. Parents should also watch their children for signs of respiratory distress between coughing spells, especially if the child has asthma.

☞ **Remember!!**

To repeat, any child with a cough should see a physician if:

- the child is less than six months old;

- the cough is sounds wet and mucousy;

- the child is coughing at night.

Will any over-the-counter (OTC) medicines help with cough?

Dr. Kelkar: Two types of cough medications are available without prescription: *antitussives* and *expectorants*. Antitussives (such as dextromethorphan) help suppress cough by blocking the cough reflex. Expectorants or *mucolytics* (such as guaifenesin) help thin mucus so the cough can get rid of thick accumulations. Some medications combine these two products. However, recent guidelines from the American College of Chest Physicians say that OTC cough medicines don't work very well and can be dangerous for children.

The Food and Drug Administration (FDA) now says cough and cold medicines should not be used in children under the age of four.

Cough and cold medicines can be dangerous for people of all ages if used incorrectly. While pharmacies now restrict the sale of cold medicines that contain pseudoephedrine or ephedrine, which can be used to make methamphetamine, experts also warn that dextromethorphan is a problem. Numerous studies by The Partnership for a Drug-Free America and others show increasing numbers of young people are using this easily available cough suppressant to get high (www.drugfree.org/Parent/Resources/Cough _Medicine_Abuse).

Are there any "home remedies" patients can use to relieve cough symptoms until they can see a doctor?

Dr. Kelkar: Home treatments can be tried but should never take the place of consulting your healthcare provider. Some things that might help you feel better include:

- drinking adequate hot/warm liquids, which can soothe the throat, help keep the body hydrated and thin mucus;

- using a cool mist humidifier in the patient's room;

- avoiding carbonated or citrus drinks, which can sometimes irritate the throat and lead to more coughing;

- following asthma medication regimens and action plans, as well as monitoring progress;

- using cough drops to soothe sore throats (for older children and adults only; they are a choking hazard for young children).

Talk with your physician before using any herbal remedies. Although some herbs are harmless, it is better to consult your doctor before trying them out.

Chapter 46

The September Epidemic:
The Back-To-School Season And Asthma

In this chapter, we discuss some things to think about as families go back to school in terms of asthma. One is the increase in asthma exacerbations during this period, and the other some thoughts about asthma control as kids go back to school.

Asthma Gets Worse In September

For several years, doctors and patients have observed that asthma control, including asthma exacerbations, increase in September. Some doctors and scientists have even called the increase in hospitalizations for asthma the "September Epidemic."

The reason for this remained obscure until recent studies that looked into the major causes of worsening asthma control and if they changed in September. It turns out that the increase in asthma worsening and kids going back to school are not merely coincidences. A detailed study of asthma attacks looking at many individuals (using 12 years of hospitalization data from the Canadian health ministry) showed that there is a sharp spike in

About This Chapter: "Asthma and the September Epidemic" was written by Dr. Fred Little for The HealthCentral Network, Inc. and first published on HealthCentral's asthma website www.MyAsthmaCentral.com, September 12, 2008. Copyright © 2008 The HealthCentral Network, Inc. All Rights Reserved.

asthma hospitalization in children about two weeks after Labor Day, the usual time of school return after summer vacation.

Even more interesting was the fact that asthma exacerbations were also increased in adults, not just children. Of note, this increase occurred about a week later than in children.

So, What Is The Connection?

It is well known that respiratory viral infections, especially a common cold virus called *rhinovirus*, are significant causes of asthma exacerbations. A parallel study to the one above demonstrated that nearly two thirds of children seeking emergency care for asthma had common cold virus in their noses. This suggests that the September Epidemic is largely caused by cold viruses. In addition, the delay in asthma exacerbations in adults suggests that children, upon returning to school, are sharing colds and cold viruses that they bring to school after summer vacation, causing a rise in colds and a rise in asthma exacerbations. These colds are then brought home and affect parents with asthma.

☞ **Remember!!**

An Interesting Aside: The study mentioned in this chapter examined a control group of asthmatics during the same time in September but whose asthma was not in a flare. The researchers found that the children without exacerbations were more likely to be taking anti-inflammatory controller medications than the children whose asthma had flared. This makes another point about long-term asthma control that is especially important going back to school:

- All asthmatics should be taking their regularly scheduled controller medicine whether their asthma is controlled or not.

Other Considerations About Asthma During School Return

The return to school is a time when many kids go back to participating in organized sports. For kids with asthma, it is an important time to be prepared. Many children have asthma that is brought on by exercise, and September and October are peak seasons for ragweed pollen in many areas of the United States. As school-age children (and college students) get back to the routine of regular exercise, it is especially important that they are taking their controller medications regularly, if directed by their asthma care provider. Asthmatics that have symptoms brought on by exercise can often minimize symptoms with exercise with premedication, say taking two puffs of albuterol 15 to 30 minutes before strenuous exercise.

Younger children may need to have their parents work with the school nurse so that asthma medications are readily available in case quick relief is needed. Ask your asthma care provider to provide an extra prescription for quick-relief medication to be kept with the school nurse or health office, so that it is available if a child runs out or forgets to keep it handy. For children who have severe allergies to foods or bees, an EpiPen should be kept with the school nurse in case of a reaction.

Schools all have different policies about keeping medications and different systems to care for kids when they are sick in school. Parents should check with their child's school to become familiar with what they have in place and how they can work with them to keep their child's asthma under the best control in school as they do at home.

Chapter 47

Managing Asthma In The School Environment

Many indoor air quality problems in schools can impact the health of students and staff, including those with asthma. Some of the indoor air quality problems include: chemical pollutants from building or building maintenance materials; chemical pollutants from science and art classes; improperly maintained ventilation systems; and allergens from classroom animals and cockroaches or pests.

Mold growth may result from standing water in maintenance rooms and near piping, or from excess moisture in ceiling tiles, carpets, and other furnishings. Also, outdoor air pollutants and pollens may enter the school through ventilation systems and/or open doors and windows.

Control Animal Allergens

Classes may commonly adopt animals as a classroom pet or science project. School staff may not realize that any warm-blooded animals including gerbils, birds, cats, dogs, mice, and rats may trigger asthma. Proteins which act as allergens in the dander, urine, or saliva of warm-blooded animals may sensitize individuals and can cause allergic reactions or trigger asthma episodes in people sensitive to animal allergens.

About This Chapter: Text in this chapter is from "Managing Asthma in the School Environment," U.S. Environmental Protection Agency (www.epa.gov), 2008.

Common Sources Found In School Settings

The most common, obvious source of animal allergen is having a pet in the classroom or school. If an animal is present in the school, there is a possibility of direct, daily exposure to the animal's dander and bodily fluids. It is important to realize that, even after extensive cleaning, pet allergen levels may stay in the indoor environment for several months after the animal is removed.

The most effective method of controlling exposure to animal allergens in schools is to keep your school free of feathered or furred animals. However, for some individuals, isolation measures may be sufficiently effective. Isolation measures include: keeping animals in localized areas; keeping animals away from upholstered furniture, carpets, and stuffed toys; and keeping sensitive individuals away from animals as much as possible.

For schools with animals, it is important to make sure that classrooms containing animals are frequently and thoroughly cleaned. In addition, animal allergens can readily migrate to other areas of the school environment through the air and on children who handle pets. Therefore, the entire building should be cleaned thoroughly.

Schools are sometimes advised to use air cleaners. Although properly used and maintained air cleaners may be effective for reducing animal dander in small areas, they should only be considered as an addition to other control methods. It is also important to carefully review information on the type of air cleaner used to make sure it is suitably sized and has high particle removal efficiency. In addition, some air-cleaning devices marketed as air purifiers emit ozone, which may be harmful to people with asthma.

Suggestions For Reducing Exposures In Schools

Remove animals from the school, if possible. If completely removing animals from the school is not possible, then try the following:

- Keep animals in cages or localized areas as much as possible; do not let them roam.

- Clean cages regularly. Consider using disposable gloves when cleaning.

- Locate animals away from ventilation system vents to avoid circulating allergens throughout the room or building.

- Locate sensitive students as far away from animals and habitats as possible.

- Keep animals away from upholstered furniture, carpets, and stuffed toys.

Clean Up Mold And Control Moisture

Molds can be found almost anywhere and they can grow on virtually any substance, providing moisture is present. Outdoors, many molds live in the soil and play a key role in the breakdown of leaves, wood, and other plant debris. Without molds we would be struggling with large amounts of dead plant matter.

Molds produce tiny spores to reproduce. Mold spores travel through the indoor and outdoor air continually. When mold spores land on a damp spot indoors, they may begin growing and digesting whatever they are growing on in order to survive. There are molds that can grow on wood, paper, carpet, and foods. If excessive moisture or water accumulates indoors, extensive mold growth may occur, particularly if the moisture problem remains undiscovered or unaddressed. There is no practical way to eliminate all mold and mold spores in the indoor environment—the way to control indoor mold growth is to control moisture. If mold is a problem in your school, you must clean up the mold and eliminate sources of moisture.

✤ It's A Fact!!

When mold growth occurs in buildings, it may be followed by reports of health symptoms from some building occupants, particularly those with allergies or respiratory problems. Potential health effects and symptoms associated with mold exposures include allergic reactions, asthma, and other respiratory complaints.

Common Moisture Sources Found In Schools

Moisture problems in school buildings can be caused by a variety of conditions, including roof and plumbing leaks, condensation, and excess humidity. Some moisture problems in schools have been linked to changes in building construction practices during the past twenty to thirty years. These changes have resulted in more tightly sealed buildings that may not allow moisture to escape easily. Moisture problems in schools are also associated with delayed maintenance or insufficient maintenance, due to budget and other constraints.

♣ It's A Fact!!
How Asthma-Friendly Is Your School?

Students with asthma need proper support at school to keep their asthma under control and be fully active. Use this checklist to find out how well your school serves students with asthma:

- Are the school buildings and grounds free of tobacco smoke at all times? Are all school buses, vans, and trucks free of tobacco smoke? Are all school events, like field trips and team games (both "at-home" and "away"), free from tobacco smoke?

- Does your school have a policy or rule that allows students to carry and use their own asthma medicines? If some students do not carry their asthma medicines, do they have quick and easy access to their medicines?

- Does your school have a written emergency plan for teachers and staff to follow to take care of a student who has an asthma attack? In an emergency, such as a fire, weather, or lockdown, or if a student forgets their medicine, does your school have standing orders and quick-relief medicines for students to use?

- Do all students with asthma have updated asthma action plans on file at the school? An asthma action plan is a written plan from the student's doctor to help manage asthma and prevent asthma attacks.

- Is there a school nurse in your school building during all school hours? Does a nurse identify, assess, and monitor students with asthma at your school? Does he or she help students with their medicines, and help them be active in physical education, sports, recess, and field trips? If a

Temporary structures in schools, such as trailers and portable classrooms, have frequently been associated with moisture and mold problems.

Suggestions For Reducing Mold Growth In Schools

Reduce indoor humidity using the following methods:

- Vent showers and other moisture-generating sources to the outside.
- Control humidity levels and dampness by using air conditioners and de-humidifiers.

school nurse is not full-time in your school, is a nurse regularly available to write plans and give the school guidance on these issues?

- Does the school nurse or other asthma education expert teach school staff about asthma, asthma action plans, and asthma medicines? Does someone teach all students about asthma and how to help a classmate who has asthma?

- Can students with asthma fully and safely join in physical education, sports, recess, and field trips? Are students' medicines nearby, before and after they exercise? Can students with asthma choose a physical activity that is different from others in the class when it is medically necessary? Can they choose another activity without fear of being ridiculed or receiving reduced grades?

- Does the school have good indoor air quality? Does the school help to reduce or prevent students' contact with allergens or irritants, indoors and outdoors, that can make their asthma worse? Allergens and irritants include tobacco smoke, pollens, animal dander, mold, dust mites, cockroaches, and strong odors or fumes from things like bug spray, paint, perfumes, and cleaners. Does the school exclude animals with fur?

If the answer to any question is "no," then it may be harder for students to have good control of their asthma. Uncontrolled asthma can hinder a student's attendance, participation, and progress in school. School staff, healthcare providers, and families should work together to make schools more asthma-friendly to promote student health and education.

Source: National Heart, Lung and Blood Institute (www.nhlbi.nih.gov), October 2008.

- Provide adequate ventilation to maintain indoor humidity levels between 30–60 percent.

- Use exhaust fans whenever cooking, dishwashing, and cleaning in food service areas.

Inspect buildings for signs of mold, moisture, leaks, or spills:

- Check for moldy odors.

- Look for water stains or discoloration on the ceiling, walls, floors, and window sills.

- Look around and under sinks for standing water, water stains, or mold.

- Inspect bathrooms for standing water, water stains, or mold.

- Do not let water stand in air conditioning or refrigerator drip pans.

Respond promptly when you see signs of moisture and/or mold, or when leaks or spills occur:

- Clean and dry any damp or wet building materials and furnishings within 24–48 hours of occurrence to prevent mold growth.

- Fix the source of the water problem or leak to prevent mold growth.

- Clean mold off hard surfaces with water and detergent, and dry completely.

Absorbent materials such as ceiling tiles, that are moldy, may need to be replaced.

- Check the mechanical room and roof for unsanitary conditions, leaks, or spills.

Prevent moisture condensation using the following methods:

- Reduce the potential for condensation on cold surfaces (e.g., windows, piping, exterior walls, roof, or floors) by adding insulation.

- For floor and carpet cleaning, remove spots and stains immediately, using the flooring manufacturer's recommended techniques. Use care to prevent excess moisture or cleaning residue accumulation and ensure that cleaned areas are dried quickly.

- In areas where there is a perpetual moisture problem, do not install carpeting (e.g., by drinking fountains, by classroom sinks, or on concrete floors with leaks or frequent condensation).

Control Cockroach And Pest Allergens

Cockroach allergens may play a significant role in asthma throughout inner-city, suburban, and rural schools. Certain proteins which act as allergens in the waste products and saliva of cockroaches can cause allergic reactions or trigger asthma symptoms in some individuals.

Pest allergens are a significant cause of occupational asthma symptoms among laboratory workers, such as scientists who work with animals in scientific investigations. These allergens may also contribute to allergies and asthma in the general population.

Common Sources Found In School Settings

Cockroaches and other pests, such as rats and mice, are often found in the school setting. Allergens from these pests may be significant asthma triggers for students and staff in schools. Pest problems in schools may be caused or worsened by a variety of conditions such as plumbing leaks, moisture problems, and improper food handling and storage practices. In order to manage a pest problem, water and food sources need to be controlled in the school environment. Therefore, it is important to avoid exposure to these allergens through the use of common sense, Integrated Pest Management (IPM) practices throughout the entire school.

There are four key IPM methods for reducing exposure to pests in the school setting:

1. Look for signs of pests.

2. Do not leave food, water, or garbage exposed.

3. Remove pest pathways and shelters.

4. Use pest control products such as poison baits, traps, and pesticide sprays, as needed.

Eliminate Secondhand Smoke Exposure

Secondhand smoke is the smoke from the burning end of a cigarette, pipe, or cigar and the smoke breathed out by a smoker. Secondhand smoke exposure causes a number of serious health effects in young children, such as coughing and wheezing, bronchitis and pneumonia, ear infections, reduced lung function, and worsened asthma attacks. Secondhand smoke is an irritant which may trigger an asthma episode, and increasing evidence suggests secondhand smoke may cause asthma in children. The Environmental Protection Agency estimates that between 200,000 and 1,000,000 children with asthma have their condition made worse by exposure to secondhand smoke. Secondhand smoke can also lead to buildup of fluid in the middle ear, the most common cause of children being hospitalized for an operation.

Common Sources Found In School Settings

The majority of schools in the United States prohibit smoking on school grounds. However, often times smoking occurs in school bathrooms, lounges, and on school grounds. This may cause problems for students and staff who have asthma.

It is important to enforce smoking bans on school grounds in order to prevent exposure from secondhand smoke. If smoking occurs within the building, secondhand smoke can travel through the ventilation system to the entire school. Also, even when people smoke outside, secondhand smoke may enter the school through the ventilation system, open windows, and doors.

To reduce secondhand smoke exposure in schools, smoking bans must be enforced on school property.

Reduce Exposure To Dust Mites

Dust mite allergens play a significant role in asthma. These allergens may cause an allergic reaction or trigger an asthma episode in sensitive individuals. In addition, there is evidence that dust mites cause new cases of asthma in susceptible children.

Dust mites are too small to be seen but are found in homes, schools, and other buildings throughout the United States. Dust mites live in mattresses, pillows, carpets, fabric-covered furniture, bedcovers, clothes, and stuffed toys. Their food source is dead skin flakes.

Common Sources Found In Schools

Dust mites may be found in schools in carpeting, upholstered furniture, stuffed animals or toys, and pillows. Stuffed animals or toys, as well as pillows for taking naps, are used mostly in the primary grades.

Suggestions for reducing exposure to dust mites in schools include the following:

- Choose washable stuffed toys and wash them often in hot water.

- Cover pillows in dust-proof (allergen-impermeable), zipped covers.

- Remove dust from hard surfaces often with a damp cloth, and vacuum carpeting and fabric-covered furniture to reduce dust buildup. Allergic people should leave the area being vacuumed. Vacuums with high efficiency filters or central vacuums may be helpful.

Chapter 48

Good Health Habits And Asthma

Your teenage years are about more than homework and driver education training: It's a critical time for building strong bones. We develop about one-half of our lifelong bone mass—not just length—in our teen years.

Our bones are constantly growing and redissolving. During the first 20 years of our lives, the emphasis is on growing bone mass. After age 30 or so, we begin to lose bone mass at a steady rate. The good news is that with proper nutrition and exercise we can slow down this bone loss. In addition, the more bone mass we've stored up as teenagers, the more we have to draw on as adults.

Teens with asthma, food allergies, or related conditions may need to take extra steps to build strong bones if they take certain medications or have restricted diets. For instance, long-term use of oral or inhaled corticosteroids may be harmful to your bones, which is one reason doctors prescribe them at the lowest possible dose. Long-term use of medications for gastroesophageal reflux disease (GERD) can hurt your body's ability to use minerals like calcium and magnesium. Children who can't eat dairy products or seafood may be missing out on bone-building nutrients, but these can be replaced with smart food choices.

About This Chapter: Text in this chapter is from "Good Food and Lots of Play: Health Habits Your Family Can Live With," © 2009 Allergy and Asthma Network Mothers of Asthmatics (www.aanma.org). All rights reserved. Reprinted with permission.

Need Those Nutrients

Calcium and vitamin D top the charts of bone-building staples. And they need each other to work effectively.

Calcium, a required mineral for healthy bones, teeth, and overall body function, can be found in dairy products, leafy green vegetables and specially fortified foods. It's not much good, though, without vitamin D, which helps the body absorb calcium. Consume vitamin D in dairy products, fish, and fortified cereals or let your skin do the work by getting 10–15 minutes of sunshine per day.

If you are allergic to cow's milk, Susan Roselle, MS, a certified nutrition specialist in Fairfax, Virginia, recommends dairy-free alternatives such as soy and rice milk (fortified with vitamin D). If you are lactose intolerant, choose lactose-free products. These products are all readily available in grocery stores.

☞ Remember!!
Calculating Calcium

Preteens and teens (ages nine to 17) should get about 1300 mg of calcium a day, according to U.S. dietary guidelines. That's a bit more than the adult recommendation (1,000 mg for ages 18–50) and significantly more than children's levels (210–270 mg for infants; 500 mg for kids ages one to three; 800 mg for ages four to eight).

How do you know if you are reaching these levels? Check food labels carefully.

Food labels list calcium content as a "percent of Daily Value (DV)." Since this is based on the adult recommendation of 1,000 mg per day, you'll have to do some simple math to figure exactly how much calcium is in each serving. To convert DV to milligrams, simply multiply by 10 or add a zero. For example, if a yogurt container lists 20% DV for calcium, multiply by 10 or add a zero and you get 200 mg of calcium for the container of yogurt.

Source: © 2009 Allergy and Asthma Network
Mothers of Asthmatics.

Where To Find Vitamin D

Vitamin D is a bit easier to calculate since the daily requirement for everyone up to age 50 is 200 mg (requirements increase for older adults). If you can't eat dairy products or fortified foods, the easiest way to get vitamin D is by exposing your skin to sunshine—just a few short minutes a day without sun block is enough to produce your body's daily requirement of vitamin D, according to Roselle. In the summer, she says, the safest times to catch those rays are before 10 a.m. or after 3:30 p.m.

Another alternative Roselle recommends is cod liver oil: 1/2 to 1 teaspoon per day. This age-old compound contains a unique combination of essential fats with vitamins A and D that support your whole body, with extra benefits for your bones. But you don't have to spoon it in Mary Poppins-style—try cod liver oil in pearls or caps!

Food Balance

Roselle's nutrition solution is simple: eat a healthy balance of many different good-for-you foods. "There's no one magic food," she concludes. "All foods have 'magic' if we get enough variety and a balanced diet. The more food variety in your diet, the easier you'll get all the nutrients you need."

And Roselle stresses the importance of a good diet over supplement use. "Supplements make up a lack after a good diet, not the other way around," she says.

Along with calcium and vitamin D, magnesium and other trace minerals are important for building bone and can't be obtained simply by taking a supplement. Magnesium helps the calcium go to your bones instead of your kidneys, where calcium can cause kidney stones. Calcium supplements don't usually contain magnesium, so eat nuts, whole grain products, or fortified cereal to get it. People with nut allergy can substitute sunflower or pumpkin seeds.

Get Up And Get Moving!

A good diet is only half of the bone-building equation: You need exercise too. According to Stacy Eichwald King, a physical therapist and personal trainer in the Washington, DC, area, bones, like muscles, become stronger with exercise.

Lack of exercise can subtract bone mass. According to Roselle, a person starts to lose bone density just 24 hours after becoming bedridden. While that may sound extreme, it points to the dangers of an inactive lifestyle. So if you are always on the sidelines due to asthma or allergy symptoms, you could be slowly losing bone mass.

Sixty minutes of exercise per day is the current recommendation for children and teens (30 minutes per day for adults), according to "Bone Health and Osteoporosis: A Surgeon General's Report." Both children and adults tend to fall short of this goal. The report shows that "only half of all teens exercise vigorously on a regular basis, and one-fourth do not exercise at all . . . Teens who miss adding bone mass to their skeletons during these critical years never make it up."

More is better when it comes to teen bone-building. According to National Osteoporosis Foundation Clinical Director Felicia Cosman, MD, "The higher the peak level (of bone mass), the better . . . Allow for some extra bone tissue in the bone bank." She says most kids aren't hitting exercise benchmarks simply through sports programs. She advises, "Parents need to step in and make sure kids get on their feet and exercise regularly." Cosman also suggests pediatricians play a more active role in educating parents and children on the importance of exercise.

An overlooked but easy and effective exercise for all age groups is walking, according to King. Walking works all muscles by carrying body weight and working against the pull of gravity, and almost anyone can do it.

Plan For Health

Roselle, King, and Cosman all agree on the importance of eating healthy food and getting physical activity every day, regardless of age. "The key message here," says Cosman, "is that our society is not doing what is recommended in the area of diet and exercise." Adds Roselle, "Our bodies are designed to be in motion—this is true no matter what your age."

If you have asthma, allergies, or food allergies, you may need to take extra steps to achieve your exercise and nutrition goals. Work on a wish list of

♣ It's A Fact!!
Poor Diet Affects Respiratory Health Of Teenagers

New epidemiologic research on teenagers in North America shows that a diet poor in essential vitamins and minerals, and other antioxidant compounds is linked to increased risk for developing respiratory conditions including asthma and reduced lung function. The study was conducted in high school seniors in 12 communities in the U.S. and Canada. The results suggest that higher dietary intake of antioxidant and anti-inflammatory micronutrients, such as vitamins A, C, and E and omega-3 fatty acids, is linked to lower reports of cough, respiratory infections, and less-severe asthma symptoms.

Lung growth and development parallels growth in physical stature; therefore the study subjects in late adolescence were near their peak of lung function. Analysis of questionnaires showed that 33 percent of the study subjects' diets were below the USDA recommendations for fruits, vegetables, essential vitamins and minerals. One-third of the teenagers were overweight, another contributing factor for asthma; 72 percent did not take multivitamins, and 25 percent smoked. The results showed that low intake of vitamins A and C, fruits and vegetables, and omega-3 fatty acids such as those found in fish and algae, was linked to reduced lung function, increased wheeze, greater risk of asthma, and symptoms of chronic bronchitis. These risks were highest among study subjects with the poorest diets who also smoked.

This study adds to the body of knowledge that a healthy diet high in antioxidants is important for proper lung growth and development to reduce the risk of asthma as well as improve the general health of teens. The researchers conclude that snacks of fresh fruit and a simple nutritious family meal would be easy ways to helps teens consume the proper amounts of essential nutrient.

Citation: Burns JS, Dockery DW, Neas LM, Schwartz J, Coull BA, Raizenne M, Speizer FE. Low dietary nutrient intakes and respiratory health in adolescents. *Chest.* 2007 Jul; 132(1)238–45.

Source: National Institute of Environmental Health Sciences, 2007.

activities you'd like to do, then work with your medical care team on how to make those wishes a reality. Your asthma or allergy management plan is a living document that you should review with your doctor and revise as often as needed.

Food allergies shouldn't deprive you of the energy you need to be active and the essential nutrients you need to build strong bones. Consult a certified nutritionist or registered dietitian to make sure your daily diet is well rounded.

If you have special concerns about your current bone density level, talk to your doctor about a bone density screening test, which measures the amount of mineral in the bones.

Then get the whole family in on the bone-building act. Building strong bones now—and good health habits—will benefit you and your whole family for your lifetimes.

✔ Quick Tip
Weight-Bearing Exercise For Kids And Teens

Exercise helps build bone mass, and weight-bearing exercise is particularly helpful in this task. Weight-bearing exercise includes any activity in which your feet and legs carry your own weight. You can:

- walk;
- run;
- jump;
- jump rope;
- dance;
- climb stairs;
- jog;
- hike;
- skate;
- play tennis, racquetball, soccer, basketball, field hockey, volleyball, softball or baseball.

Source: © 2009 Allergy and Asthma Network Mothers of Asthmatics.

Chapter 49

Exercise And Asthma

Do you cough, wheeze, and have a tight chest or shortness of breath when you exercise? If yes, you may have exercise-induced bronchoconstriction (EIB). This happens when the tubes that bring air into and out of your lungs narrow with exercise, causing symptoms of asthma.

An estimated 300 million people worldwide suffer from asthma, according to the World Health Organization, and strenuous exercise makes it worse for many people. Some people have EIB who do not otherwise have asthma, and people with allergies may also have trouble breathing during exercise.

Symptoms: If you have EIB, you may have problems breathing within five to 20 minutes after exercise. Your symptoms may include:

- wheezing;
- tight chest;
- cough;
- shortness of breath;
- chest pain (rarely).

About This Chapter: Text in this chapter begins with information from "Exercise and Asthma," © 2009 American Academy of Allergy, Asthma, and Immunology (www.aaaai.org). Reprinted with permission. Additional information about asthma and exercise is cited separately in the chapter.

Triggers: People with EIB are very sensitive to both low temperatures and dry air. Air is usually warmed and humidified by the nose; but during demanding activity people breathe more through their mouths. This allows cold, dry air to reach the lower airways and the lungs without passing through the nose, triggering asthma symptoms. Air pollutants, high pollen levels and viral respiratory infections also may be triggers. Other causes of symptoms with exercise may be that you are out of shape, have poorly controlled nasal allergies or vocal chord issues.

Diagnosis: Wheezing or tightness in the chest can be serious, so let your physician know about your symptoms. Your doctor can help you by:

- getting your health history;
- doing a breathing test (called spirometry) at rest;
- doing a follow-up exercise challenge test.

If your breathing test shows that you might have asthma, your doctor may give you a drug to inhale such as albuterol. If your breathing test numbers improve after inhaling the medicine then the diagnosis of asthma is more likely. If your breathing test is normal, you may be asked to take an additional test, called a bronchoprovocation challenge test. Your doctor will have you exercise in your sport, run outside, or have you cycle or run on a treadmill. Before and after the exercise, your doctor will test the amount of air you force out of your lungs with a spirometry test. If you exhale air less forcefully after exercise then the problem may be EIB.

Treatment: The first step is to develop a treatment plan with your physician. EIB associated with more generalized asthma is prevented with controller medications taken regularly (such as mast cell stabilizers, inhaled steroids, and leukotriene modifiers) or by using medicines before you exercise (short-acting beta agonists such as albuterol). When EIB symptoms occur they can be treated with short-acting beta agonists.

In addition to medications, warm-ups and warm-downs may prevent or lessen EIB symptoms. Some people may want to limit exercise when they have viral infections, temperatures are low, or pollen and air pollution levels are high.

Recommended Activities: The goal of an asthma treatment plan is to keep your symptoms under control so that you can enjoy exercising or sports activities. However, there are some activities that are better for people with EIB. For instance, swimmers are exposed to warm, moist air as they exercise which does not tend to trigger asthma symptoms. Swimming also helps strengthen upper body muscles.

Walking, leisure biking and hiking are also good sporting activities for people with EIB. Team sports that require short bursts of energy, such as baseball, football, and short-term track and field are less likely to cause symptoms than sports that have a lot of ongoing activity such as soccer, basketball, field hockey or long-distance running.

Cold weather activities such as cross-country skiing and ice hockey are more likely to make symptoms worse, but with proper diagnosis and treatment, many people with EIB can participate and excel in almost any sport or activity.

When To See An Allergy/Asthma Specialist: One of the first steps to controlling EIB is finding the right help. An allergist/immunologist, often referred to as an allergist, is an internist or pediatrician with at least two years of advanced training in allergic diseases. An allergist can help figure out the cause of your symptoms and develop a treatment plan that can keep you exercising. You should see an allergist/immunologist if you:

✔ Quick Tip
Healthy Tips

- If you cough, wheeze, and have a tight chest or shortness of breath when you exercise you could have EIB.

- Walking, leisure biking, swimming, and hiking are good sporting activities for people with EIB.

- Cold weather activities such as cross-country skiing and ice hockey as well as sports that require short bursts of high energy are more likely to make symptoms worse.

- An allergist/immunologist can help figure out the cause of your symptoms and develop a treatment plan that can keep you exercising.

Source: © 2009 American Academy of Allergy, Asthma, and Immunology.

- have exercise-induced symptoms that are unusual or do not respond well to treatment;

- have had exercise-induced anaphylaxis or food-dependent exercise-induced anaphylaxis;

- have a history of asthma and want to scuba dive.

Asthma And Exercise

From the Global Strategy for Asthma Management and Prevention, Global Initiative for Asthma (GINA) 2008. Available from: http://www.ginasthma.org.

Is it good for people with asthma to exercise?

Yes. Even though physical exercise is a common trigger of asthma symptoms, it is just as important for people with asthma to exercise as for anyone

☞ **Remember!!**
How can I avoid exercise-induced asthma?

The best way to avoid exercise-induced asthma is to make sure that your asthma is properly controlled and, if necessary, that you take extra medication before exercising. A good warm-up also reduces the risk of exercise-induced asthma.

Anti-inflammatory treatment, preferably with inhaled corticosteroids, taken regularly will prevent exercise-induced asthma in many people. However, some people still need to take an airway opener (bronchodilator) before exercise. Many people with asthma should have daily treatment with both inhaled corticosteroids and a long-acting airway opener. Combination medications are now available in many countries.

Particular types of exercise, such as running and jogging, are more likely to expose the airways to large volumes of dry air and trigger asthma, while less vigorous activities, like swimming and yoga, are less likely to cause these symptoms.

Source: © 2008 Global Initiative for Asthma (GINA).

else. Keep in mind that it takes time to get in shape and you lose fitness quickly when you stop exercising regularly.

With the right medication, most people with asthma will be able to do some kind of physical exercise, many will feel no restrictions, and some will only react to exercise in combination with other triggers.

Exercise is good for you so why can it cause asthma symptoms?

The common symptoms of exercise-induced asthma are:

- wheezing;
- abnormal shortness of breath;
- tightness in the chest;
- coughing.

You may have just one of these symptoms or a combination of them. Treatment with an airway opener (reliever) medicine, such as a quick-acting bronchodilator, should immediately relieve one or more of the symptoms. If not, you should discuss other possible reasons for the symptoms with your doctor.

Are some kinds of physical activities more suitable for people with asthma?

Aerobics is an effective activity, which allows you to train in sessions at varying intensities. The purpose of aerobics is to develop your breathing and heart capacity. If you start by warming up with light jogging, you can, for example, increase the intensity for a couple of minutes, slow down again and then increase the speed once more.

Indoor swimming is also thought to be good exercise, because it takes place at a controlled temperature and in a humid environment. You can also try an aerobic approach by increasing and decreasing your swimming speed.

Whatever you do, make sure you warm up first, because this will reduce the likelihood of exercise-induced asthma.

The most important thing is that the exercise you do is fun; otherwise it is easy to skip it. It is important to find the exercise that suits you!

How intensively do I dare to exercise?

Your training program should help you get in better shape gradually. Remember that it takes time to get in shape. As a rule of thumb, you should feel fine after every training session. It is therefore important that you do not try to do too much at once. You should not feel totally exhausted for a couple of hours after every training session.

If you often get asthma symptoms when you exercise intensively, this could be a signal that you are not taking enough medication or that your asthma does not allow such intensive exercise. Talk to your doctor about your treatment to see if anything can be done.

I often feel my asthma when I jog. Do I have to quit jogging?

Absolutely not! Very often, just preparing yourself for jogging somewhat differently can be enough. There are two things you should remember. First, take your airway opener medication about 15 minutes before you start. Secondly, warm up properly before you go full steam ahead.

What should I do if I get asthma symptoms while exercising?

Make sure that you always carry a quick-relief airway opener medication and use it promptly if necessary.

If exercising often causes asthma symptoms, you may need to take a better preventive medication, or to avoid a particular kind of exercise.

Can I take asthma medications and still take part in competitive sports?

Yes. Most of the commonly prescribed asthma medications are allowed in competitive sports. Generally, the use of inhaled anti-inflammatory medicines and some bronchodilators is allowed, but corticosteroids in tablet, syrup, suppository, or injectable form are banned.

Check with your doctor or the national sports associations, especially if competing internationally, to be sure that your medication does not violate any doping rules. In some cases, you will need a certificate from your doctor about your need for asthma medication.

Chapter 50

Teen Smoking And Asthma

Smoking And Asthma

You may have family photo albums full of people smoking at every type of event, from birthday parties to company picnics. That's because smoking was once accepted pretty much everywhere—even in doctor's offices. But that changed as we learned more about the health problems it causes.

If you have asthma, smoking is especially risky because of the damage it does to the lungs.

When someone smokes, he or she may cough, wheeze, and feel short of breath. This is because smoke irritates the airways, causing them to become swollen, narrow, and filled with sticky mucus. These are the same things that happen during an asthma flare-up. That's why smoking can cause asthma flare-ups to happen more often. Those flare-ups may be more severe and harder to control, even with medicine.

About This Chapter: This chapter begins with "Smoking and Asthma," June 2007, reprinted with permission from www.kidshealth.org. Copyright © 2007 The Nemours Foundation. This information was provided by KidsHealth, one of the largest resources online for medically reviewed health information written for parents, kids, and teens. For more articles like this one, visit www.KidsHealth.org, or www.TeensHealth.org. Additional information about quitting smoking is cited separately within the chapter.

If You Smoke

You may have started smoking be-cause all your friends do or because you grew up in a house where lots of people smoked. Some people try smoking because they are curious or bored. No matter why you started, if you're thinking about quitting, it would probably help your asthma.

♣ **It's A Fact!!**

If you smoke, you aren't alone. Ninety percent of smokers start be-fore they are 21. And many of them keep smoking because it is a highly addictive habit.

Source: © 2007 The Nemours Foundation.

Smoking can undo the effect of any con-troller medicine you're taking. It also can force you to use your rescue medicine more often. It can also disturb your sleep by making you cough more at night and can affect how well you perform in sports or other physical activities. Worst of all, it can send you to the emer-gency department with a severe asthma flare-up.

If you decide to quit smoking, you don't have to go it alone. Seek the sup-port of others who are also trying to quit. You also might ask your doctor about medication or different strategies that can help you crave cigarettes less.

If Other People Smoke

Even if you don't smoke, you may still run into smoky situations in res-taurants, parties, or even at home if one of your family members smokes. Secondhand smoke is a known asthma trigger, so you'll want to avoid it as much as possible if you have asthma.

If you hang out with smokers or have a family member who smokes in the house, you are likely to have more frequent and severe asthma symp-toms. You may have to take more medicine and your asthma may be harder to control. Finally, you may find yourself at the doctor's office or emergency department more often because of asthma symptoms.

There's not much you can do about other people's behavior, but you should let your friends and family know that what they are doing is mak-ing your asthma worse. Ask them not to smoke in your house or car. It's your air, after all.

How Can I Quit Smoking?

First, congratulate yourself. Just reading this article is a huge step toward becoming tobacco free. Many people don't quit smoking because they think it's too hard to do. They think they'll quit someday.

It's true, for most people quitting isn't easy. After all, the nicotine in cigarettes is a powerfully addictive drug. But with the right approach, you can overcome the cravings.

The Difficulty In Kicking The Habit

Smokers may have started smoking because their friends did or because it seemed cool. But they keep on smoking because they became addicted to nicotine, one of the chemicals in cigarettes and smokeless tobacco. Nicotine is both a stimulant and a depressant. That means nicotine increases the heart rate at first and makes people feel more alert (like caffeine, another stimulant). Then it causes depression and fatigue. The depression and fatigue—and the drug withdrawal from nicotine—make people crave another cigarette to perk up again. According to many experts, the nicotine in tobacco is as addictive as cocaine or heroin.

But don't be discouraged; millions of Americans have permanently quit smoking. These strategies can help you quit, too:

Put It In Writing: People who want to make a change often are more successful when they put it in writing. So write down all the reasons why you want to quit smoking, such as the money you will save or the stamina you'll gain for playing sports. Keep that list where you can see it, and add to it as you think of new reasons.

Get Support: People whose friends and family help them quit are much more likely to succeed. If you don't want to tell your parents or family that you smoke, make sure your friends know, and consider confiding in a counselor or other adult you trust. And if you're having a hard time finding people to support you (if, say, all your friends smoke and none of them is interested in quitting), you might consider joining a support group, either in person or online.

Strategies That Work

Set A Quit Date: Pick a day that you'll stop smoking. Tell your friends (and your family, if they know you smoke) that you're going to quit smoking on that day. Just think of that day as a dividing line between the smoking you and the new and improved nonsmoker you'll become. Mark it on your calendar.

Throw Away Your Cigarettes—All Of Your Cigarettes: People can't stop smoking with cigarettes still around to tempt them. Even toss out that emergency pack you have stashed in the secret pocket of your backpack. Get rid of your ashtrays and lighters, too.

Wash All Your Clothes: Get rid of the smell of cigarettes as much as you can by washing all your clothes and having your coats or sweaters dry-cleaned. If you smoked in your car, clean that out, too.

Think About Your Triggers: You're probably aware of the situations when you tend to smoke, such as after meals, when you're at your best friend's house, while drinking coffee, or as you're driving. These situations are your triggers for smoking—it feels automatic to have a cigarette when you're in them. Once you've figured out your triggers, try these tips:

- Avoid these situations. For example, if you smoke when you drive, get a ride to school, walk, or take the bus for a few weeks. If you normally smoke after meals, make it a point to do something else after you eat, like read or call a friend.

- Change the place. If you and your friends usually smoke in restaurants or get takeout and eat in the car, suggest that you sit in the no-smoking section the next time you go out to eat.

- Substitute something else for cigarettes. It can be hard to get used to not holding something and having something in your mouth. If you have this problem, stock up on carrot sticks, sugar-free gum, mints, toothpicks, or even lollipops.

Physical And Mental Effects

Expect some physical symptoms. If you smoke regularly, you're probably physically addicted to nicotine and your body may experience some symptoms of withdrawal when you quit. These may include:

* headaches or stomachaches;

* crabbiness, jumpiness, or depression;

* lack of energy;

* dry mouth or sore throat;

* desire to pig out.

☞ Remember!!
Slip-Ups Happen

If you slip up, don't give up! Major changes sometimes have false starts. If you're like many people, you may quit successfully for weeks or even months and then suddenly have a craving that's so strong you feel like you have to give in. Or maybe you accidentally find yourself in one of your trigger situations and give in to temptation. If you slip up, it doesn't mean you've failed, it just means you're human. Here are some ways to get back on track:

* Think about your slip as one mistake. Take notice of when and why it happened and move on.

* Did you become a heavy smoker after one cigarette? We didn't think so—it happened more gradually, over time. Keep in mind that one cigarette didn't make you a smoker to start with, so smoking one cigarette (or even two or three) after you've quit doesn't make you a smoker again.

* Remind yourself why you've quit and how well you've done—or have someone in your support group, family, or friends do this for you.

Reward yourself. As you already know, quitting smoking isn't easy. Give yourself a well-deserved reward! Set aside the money you usually spend on cigarettes. When you've stayed tobacco free for a week, two weeks, or a month, buy yourself a treat like a new CD, book, movie, or some clothes. And every smoke-free year, celebrate again. You earned it.

Source: © 2006 The Nemours Foundation

Luckily, the symptoms of nicotine withdrawal will pass—so be patient. Try not to give in and sneak a smoke because you'll just have to deal with the symptoms longer.

Keep yourself busy. Many people find it's best to quit on a Monday, when they have school or work to keep them busy. The more distracted you are, the less likely you'll be to crave cigarettes. Staying active is also a good way to make sure you keep your weight down and your energy up, even as you're experiencing the symptoms of nicotine withdrawal.

Quit gradually. Some people find that gradually decreasing the number of cigarettes they smoke each day is an effective way to quit. However, this strategy doesn't work for everyone—you may find you have to stop completely at once. This is known as quitting "cold turkey."

Use a nicotine replacement if you need to. If you find that none of these strategies is working, you might talk to your doctor about treatments. Using a nicotine replacement, such as gum, patches, inhalers, or nasal sprays, can be very helpful. Sprays and inhalers are available by prescription only, and it's important to see your doctor before buying the patch and gum over the counter. That way, your doctor can help you find the solution that will work best for you. For example, the patch requires the least effort on your part, but it doesn't offer the almost instantaneous nicotine kick that gum does.

Chapter 51

Traveling With Asthma

The fun of traveling is being in a completely different place. But if you have asthma, a new environment can seem less fun because there's always the worry that something unexpected may cause an asthma flare-up. But you can take steps to help avoid problems while you're away from home—so you can concentrate on the fun.

Before You Go

Before you leave, make sure your asthma is well controlled. If it has been flaring up, check with your doctor before you head off on your trip. He or she may need to adjust your medicine or ask you to come in for a visit.

When packing, remember all medicine you're taking for your asthma, including rescue and controller medicines. Keep your medications in your carry-on bags so they're always with you. It's also a good idea to pack a little extra medication, so you don't run out while you're on the road.

About This Chapter: This chapter begins with text from "Traveling and Asthma," June 2007, reprinted with permission from www.kidshealth.org. Copyright © 2007 The Nemours Foundation. This information was provided by KidsHealth, one of the largest resources online for medically reviewed health information written for parents, kids, and teens. For more articles like this one, visit www.KidsHealth.org, or www.TeensHealth.org. Additional information about traveling with asthma is cited separately within the chapter.

If you'll be leaving the country, it can help to have a letter from your doctor that describes your asthma and your medicines. This can help you with airport security or customs. You also might want to know the generic names of your medicines. These are the chemical names of the medicine, not the brand name the drug company has given it. If you need to get a refill in another country, the medication might have a different brand name. You can get the generic names from your doctor's office or pharmacist.

Other things to pack include your peak flow meter (if you use one), a copy of your asthma action plan, your health insurance card, and your doctor's phone number.

Windows Up Or Down?

Trains, buses, and even your family car might have dust mites and mold trapped in the upholstery or the ventilation system. You can't do much about a bus or train (except make sure you've taken your controller medication and have your rescue medication handy). But if you're traveling by car, ask the driver to run the air conditioner or heater with the windows open for at least 10 minutes. If pollen or air pollution trigger your asthma and counts are high during your trip, travel with the windows closed and the air conditioner on.

Finding The Friendly Skies

All flights within the United States are smoke free, but some international flights are not. If you find yourself on one of these flights, ask to be seated as far from the smoking section as possible. The air on planes is also very dry, and this can trigger an asthma flare-up. Make sure you have your rescue medications handy and try to drink a lot of water.

Home Away From Home

If you're staying in a hotel, you may find that something in the room triggers your asthma. Requesting a sunny, dry room away from the hotel's pool might help. If animal allergens trigger your asthma, ask for a room that has never had pets in it. And you should always stay in a nonsmoking room.

If it's possible, bringing your own blanket and pillow can help prevent a flare-up.

If you're staying with family or friends, tell them in advance about your triggers. They won't be able to clear away all dust mites or mold, but they can dust and vacuum carefully, especially in the room you'll sleep in. You also can ask them to avoid using scented candles, potpourri, or aerosol products, if those bother you.

Just like at home, you'll want to avoid tobacco smoke. Ask anyone who smokes to step outside, especially if you're sharing a room. Wood fires in the fireplace or woodstove also could be a problem for you.

Traveling On Your Own

If possible, carry a copy of your asthma action plan so people who are traveling with you (or the people you're staying with) can help if you have any breathing trouble. If you don't have a copy of your plan, let these people know which medicines you take, what the dosages are, and the number where your parents and your doctor can be reached, in case of an emergency.

Without your parents along, you will have more responsibility for your asthma. Keep your triggers in mind and take steps to avoid them. If pollen bothers you, find out what the readings are on a day when you'll be going for a hike or taking part in other outdoor activities. If air pollution bothers you, make sure you keep that in mind when you're visiting a smoggy city. Cities like Los Angeles make information on air pollution levels available through their weather services.

If you're planning to take part in any new activities while you're away, talk to your doctor about them before you leave. And whatever you do, make sure your rescue medication is nearby in case you need it.

Of course, you'll want to forget about your asthma and have fun while you're away. And the best way to do this is by planning ahead and having your medication with you—so you don't have to worry if you do have a flare-up. If you ignore your asthma completely by not taking precautions, there's a chance you could end up in the emergency department. And that's no way to spend a vacation.

Ensuring Health Care Availability On Vacation

Check the extent and limitations of your medical insurance policies before leaving the country or your state. Know in advance if your plan or group will cover physician and hospital visits away from its operating territories.

When you know your vacation destination, get recommendations from your physician for asthma and allergy specialists in that area, or contact the local state medical society at the destination for recommendations on area specialists. In relatively populated areas, ask for several potential healthcare providers, to allow for comparisons.

You can also write, call or visit the web sites of the following organizations:

American Academy of Allergy, Asthma and Immunology
611 East Wells Street
Milwaukee, WI 53202
800-822-2762
Website: www.aaaai.org

American College of Allergy, Asthma and Immunology
85 W. Algonquin Road, Suite 550
Arlington, IL 60005
800-842-7777
Website: www.allergy.mcg.edu

If your vacation takes you to a foreign land, you might consider contacting the International Association for Medical Assistance to Travelers. For a low-cost donation to this nonprofit organization, you can receive a directory of English-speaking physicians worldwide who have trained in either the United States, Canada, or the United Kingdom. It can also provide forms for your own clinical records, immunization information for specific countries and worldwide climate charts. For further details call:

IAMAT

417 Center Street
Lewiston, NY, 14092
Phone: 716-754-4883

☞ **Remember!!**
Sensible Behaviors And Actions

- During the hot weather season, people with asthma and allergies should drink plenty of fluids.

- Avoid exposure to tobacco smoke whenever possible.

- Call ahead to order a special meal on the airplane. Or pack your own "safe" snacks.

- When eating out, ask the waiter if sulfites have been used as a food preservative. If so, find out whether special preparations without sulfite additives can be ordered. If eating out in a country where you don't speak the language, have a warning note drafted in the local language that alerts wait staff to your allergy.

- Prior to beginning a lengthy auto trip to your vacation spot, take appropriate measures to rid the vehicle's ventilating and air conditioning system of mold and mildew.

- For those prone to exercise-induced asthma, it may be a good idea to keep prescribed emergency medication on you at all times.

- Request a hotel room that is nonsmoking and mold-free.

If you have questions about the primary allergens and pollen count in the area you are visiting, contact the local Chamber of Commerce. Or you can call the National Allergy Bureau at 1-800-9-POLLEN or visit the Asthma and Allergy Foundation of America (AAFA) website. AAFA also has a national network of educational support groups. One may be in the area you are traveling to and could provide you with useful local information. Call 800-7-ASTHMA for support group contacts.

Source: © 2005 Asthma and Allergy Foundation of America.

Chapter 52

Why Nonadherence To Treatment Plans Is A Problem

Defining Nonadherence To Asthma Therapy

Assessing and understanding patient adherence in the management of asthma requires an appreciation of the diversity and complexity of adherence behavior. Adherence to medication can be defined as the degree to which use of medication by the patient corresponds with the prescribed regimen.

Patients who regularly and consistently follow the prescribed regimen demonstrate adherent use. Adherence to medication is not a dichotomy, however, and patients can demonstrate a wide variety of patterns of medication use. The efficacy of asthma therapies can be modulated by these adherence patterns in several ways.

The most obvious form of nonadherence is chronic under-use, i.e., the patient consistently uses less medication than is prescribed. Chronic under-treatment of asthma may lead to poor control of symptoms and greater reliance on *pro re nata* (PRN) treatments for the relief of acute asthma symptoms.

About This Chapter: Text in this chapter is excerpted from "Adherence to Long-Term Therapies—Evidence for Action," http://apps.who.int/medicinedocs/en/d/Js4883e/. © 2003 World Health Organization. Reprinted with permission. The complete text, including references, is available online through the World Health Organization website.

Patients may also have an erratic pattern of adherence, in which medication use alternates between fully adherent (usually when symptomatic) and under-use or total non-use (when asymptomatic). Patients with erratic adherence may present for treatment of acute asthma although they apparently adhere completely to their prescribed regimen. Some patients relying solely on inhaled beta-agonists for symptom relief may be prone to over-use during acute bronchospasm. This may cause a patient to delay seeking care, or lead to complications associated with excessive use of beta-agonists.

Patients may exhibit a different pattern of adherence to each of the various medications prescribed for the management of their asthma. For example, a patient may under-use the prescribed prophylactic anti-inflammatory ("controller" or "preventer") medications while remaining appropriately adherent to the regular taking of the beta-agonist. Adherence to an asthma action plan that outlines how and when both controller and reliever medications should be taken and when to seek urgent care has been shown to be one of the most effective forms of asthma self-management. Finally, in order for medications delivered by metered dose inhaler (MDI) to control asthma optimally, the patient must adhere to the instructions for correct MDI use, or use an MDI spacer. Although MDI adherence has rarely been assessed in clinical or research settings, those studies that have examined patterns of MDI use by patients have suggested that poor technique is widespread (resulting both from inadequate instruction and patients' forgetfulness), and that improved MDI adherence can influence asthma management.

Rates Of Adherence To Inhaled Corticosteroids And Other Drugs For The Prevention Of Asthma

Extensive research conducted in Australia, Canada, the United Kingdom, the United States and elsewhere has found that nonadherence with asthma therapy is widespread, and is a significant risk factor for asthma morbidity and mortality. Because of the limited sensitivity and specificity of self-reported measures of adherence, some of the most convincing studies have used objective measures, such as pharmacy databases, medication measurement, and electronic medication monitors to assess adherence behavior.

♣ It's A Fact!!

Conservative estimates indicate that almost half of the prescription medications dispensed yearly are not taken as prescribed. The real-life response to a clinician's prescription of preventive therapy will include a range of undesirable patient behaviors, including a failure to fill the initial prescription, erratic use or under-use of therapy, and premature discontinuation of therapy. Studies indicate that primary nonadherence (not filling initial prescriptions) ranges from 6 to 44 percent.

Even when patients fill prescriptions for asthma medications, studies of secondary nonadherence (rates of medication use) suggest that long-term rates of adherence to preventive therapies (e.g., controller or preventer medications) among adult patients are often poor. Spector et al., one of the first investigative teams to use an electronic medication monitor to examine adherence to MDI-delivered medications, followed 19 adult asthmatic patients using an anti-inflammatory drug for 12 weeks. Patients adhered to the four-times-daily regimen for a mean of 47 percent of the days, with a range of 4.3 percent to 95 percent. Patients were also asked to maintain asthma diaries as part of this study, and a comparative analysis of electronic data and diary data found that subjects over-reported their appropriate use of medication in their diaries more than 50 percent of the time. In a similar study, Mawhinney et al. studied adherence in adult asthmatic patients over a three to four week period. Adherence to the medication as prescribed was observed, on average, for 37 percent of the days, and under-use on more than 38 percent of the days monitored. Yeung et al. used an electronic monitor to follow patients' use of inhaled corticosteroids over a period of two to three weeks. When patients were aware that they were being monitored, 60 percent of them were fully adherent, 20 percent were partially adherent (taking just 70 percent of the prescribed dose) and 20 percent were totally nonadherent. However, when patients were unaware of the monitoring, six out of 11 took between 30 percent and 51 percent of the prescribed doses.

Several studies have suggested that patients from low-income, ethnic-minority groups (primarily African American) in developed countries may have lower rates of adherence to asthma therapy. Celano et al. examined adherence to anti-inflammatory medication delivered by MDI in low-income, urban, primarily African American children with asthma. Adherence to treatment administered by MDI was estimated by weighing canisters and calculating the ratio of the number of puffs used over the study period to the number of puffs prescribed. Estimated MDI adherence in this study was 44 percent for all participants and only 12 percent of the children had rates above 75 percent. In a group of 80 asthma patients, treated under the Medicaid scheme, who were repeat users of the emergency department or overnight hospitalization, only 46 percent had been prescribed ICSs (inhaled corticosteroids) and only 43 percent had a written action plan. Less than half of children with asthma living in Tennessee, receiving treatment funded by Medicaid, had a prescription for oral corticosteroids filled following an emergency department visit or a period of hospitalization for asthma.

Forms Of Nonadherence

Understanding patient nonadherence to ICS therapy requires the recognition that there are different forms of nonadherent behavior with diverse contributory factors. Careful clinical interviewing can reveal these problems and set the stage for identifying appropriate strategies for ameliorating them.

Erratic Nonadherence

Perhaps the form of nonadherence that is most common and most acknowledged by patients and providers is doses missed because of forgetfulness, changing schedules, or busy lifestyles. Patients who exhibit erratic nonadherence understand their prescribed regimen and would often like to adhere appropriately. However, they find it difficult to comply because the complexity of their lives interferes with adherence, or because they have not prioritized asthma management. Patients who have changing work schedules or chaotic lifestyles may have difficulty establishing the habit of a new medication regimen. For some patients Monday through Friday adherence presents no problem, but weekends or holidays disrupt medication routines. Strategies to improve erratic adherence center on simplification of the regimen (e.g., once-a-day dosing), establishing new habits through linking (e.g., keeping the MDI next to the toothbrush) and cues and memory aids (e.g., pill organizers).

Unwitting Nonadherence

Many patients may be inadvertently nonadherent to the prescribed therapy because they have failed to understand fully either the specifics of the regimen or the necessity for adherence. Studies have found that patients frequently forget instructions given to them by a physician during a clinic visit. MDIs, unlike pill bottles, do not usually have attached labels with dosing instructions. In asthma management it is common for patients to misunderstand the difference between PRN medication and daily medication. Or, they may interpret the prescription for "ICS twice every day" as meaning "ICS twice every day—when you have symptoms."

Intelligent Nonadherence

Sometimes patients purposely alter, discontinue, or even fail to initiate ICS therapy. This deliberate nonadherence is called intelligent nonadherence, reflecting a reasoned choice, rather than necessarily a wise one. Patients who feel better may decide that they no longer need to take prescribed medications. Fear of perceived short- or long-term side-effects of ICS may cause some patients to reduce or discontinue dosing. Patients may abandon a therapy because bad taste, complexity, or interference with daily life may

☞ Remember!!

Regardless of the reason for nonadherence to medication, the necessary first step toward addressing the problem is identifying it through effective, open-ended communication between patient and provider. Only careful interviewing and active listening will equip the provider of asthma care with the information necessary to establish and reinforce adherence to appropriate medication. The time constraints placed on clinicians by managed care represent a serious barrier to carrying out this recommendation.

convince them that the disadvantages of therapy outweigh the benefits. Patients may find that some variation of the prescribed therapy works better than that prescribed by the doctor. Given the well-documented underuse of ICS, the fact that ICS therapy is as successful in the management of asthma as it is, suggests that many patients manage quite well with altered or reduced doses. This deliberate nonadherence, like any other pattern of nonadherence, does not necessarily result in worsening asthma. In every clinical practice there are patients who have knowingly altered their prescribed therapy, yet their health professional may never discover this modification.

Conclusions

Nonadherence to regimens for asthma treatment may have several causes including inadequate knowledge and skill on the part of the patient, and inadequate awareness of the problem, or lack of skill to address it, on the part of the health professional. Patients must have a basic understanding of their illness and its treatment if we are to expect even minimal adherence. Achievement of adherence requires considerable effort from both the patient and caregiver. To perform the daily tasks necessary for successful control of their asthma, patients must be well motivated and convinced that their own behavior will result in improved health, a concept referred to as self-efficacy. Simply giving information to patients is unlikely to change behavior; health care providers must understand the psychological principles that underlie self-management training and comprehend that motivating patients requires more than informing them briefly about the prescription that has just been written. At the core of these principles is the need to establish treatment goals that can be embraced both by health professionals and patients in a partnership that requires regular and reciprocal communication.

Patients will not perform the work necessary to achieve goals they do not understand or do not view as necessary and important. Once appropriate goals have been established, most patients require assistance in determining how to evaluate their changing symptoms and how to use their written action plan to make effective decisions about daily self-management behavior.

Chapter 53

Dealing With Asthma Emergencies

How To Avoid The ER If You Have Asthma

Going to the emergency room is the last resort for someone who has asthma. If a flare-up is really out of hand—and your medicine isn't working or you forgot your inhaler—you need to get emergency care for your breathing trouble. The good news is that you can prevent emergency room visits if you take steps to get your asthma under control. Read on to find out how you can manage your asthma and avoid the ER.

Make A Plan: Work with your doctor to create a personalized plan for managing your asthma (also called an asthma action plan). This plan should be realistic and should fit into your daily life. Your plan should outline your day-to-day treatment, give you symptoms to watch for, and provide you with step-by-step instructions on what to do when you're having a flare-up.

Take Charge: Once you have a plan, use it to take control. Put any daily requirements the plan calls for—such as taking medications before

About This Chapter: This chapter begins with "How to Avoid the ER If You Have Asthma," April 2007, reprinted with permission from www.kidshealth.org. Copyright © 2007 The Nemours Foundation. This information was provided by KidsHealth, one of the largest resources online for medically reviewed health information written for parents, kids, and teens. For more articles like this one, visit www.KidsHealth.org, or www.TeensHealth.org. Additional information about asthma emergencies is cited separately in the chapter.

exercising—into your schedule so you don't forget to do these. Keep a copy of your plan with you so you'll know what to do if you have a flare-up. And don't be afraid to talk to your doctor if you find your plan isn't working for you. He or she can adjust your plan so it's more effective.

Avoid Triggers: Your doctor should be able to help you figure out the triggers that can lead you to have an asthma flare-up. These may include animals, dust mites, mold, tobacco smoke, cold air, exercise, and infections. Once you know what your triggers are, you can try to steer clear of them.

> **✔ Quick Tip**
> **When To Get Help**
>
> Sometimes people say: "Just give it time." But that approach may not work with an asthma flare-up. If you forgot your inhaler or your rescue medicine doesn't seem to be working, get emergency medical care.
>
> Source: © 2007 The Nemours Foundation.

Take Your Controller Medicine: Controller medicines work over a long period of time to prevent flare-ups. Depending on how serious your asthma is, you may have to take controller medications every day, even if you feel great. It's tempting to skip daily controller medications—lots of people fall into the trap of thinking they can just use rescue medicine when they have a flare-up. But doing this actually makes it more likely you'll have a flare-up and that it will be a severe one.

Have Your Inhaler With You: Rescue medicine can help you during a flare-up, so don't leave home without it. Many emergency room visits for asthma happen because the person forgot his or her inhaler.

Know The Early Signs Of A Flare-Up: Everyone's asthma is different. Some people cough only at night, and others might have flare-ups whenever they get a cold or exercise outside. Get to know your asthma and pay attention to what happens before you have a flare-up so that you know the early warning signs. These signs may not mean for sure that a flare-up will happen, but they can help you to plan ahead.

Peak Flow Meters

A peak flow meter can be a really useful tool in helping to determine if you might be getting ready for a flare-up. Your doctor can tell you which number ranges to watch out for.

Other early warning signs of a flare-up may include:

- coughing, even if you don't have a cold;

- tightness in your chest;

- throat clearing;

- rapid or irregular breathing;

- inability to stand or sit still;

- unusual fatigue;

- restless sleep.

Your asthma action plan should tell you how to handle any early signs of a flare-up. This may mean using your rescue medicine or adjusting your controller meds slightly.

✔ Quick Tip
Signs You May Need To Go To The ER

Even if you do your best, you may still get the occasional flare-up. Don't be embarrassed to get emergency help if you think you need it. Here are some situations that call for emergency care:

- You take your asthma medicine and your flare-up doesn't get any better.

- You feel a little better after taking your medicine, but your serious symptoms come back quickly.

- You see that your lips and fingernails are bluish or grayish.

- You have trouble talking or walking.

Source: © 2007 The Nemours Foundation.

Flare-ups do happen, of course. An important part of staying away from the ER or your doctor's office is calmly and carefully following your asthma action plan when you do have a flare-up. Most flare-ups, when treated as your doctor tells you to, will go away quickly.

If you feel comfortable doing so, you might want to let your friends know about your asthma. Then they can help you if you ever have a severe flare-up.

Although asthma can be dangerous, when it's well managed it's rarely life threatening. Studies show that on the rare occasions when people have died from asthma, it's usually because they haven't taken their medications as prescribed and they have a history of repeated severe asthma flare-ups and emergency care. If you take your asthma seriously and work to manage it, you may never need to go to the emergency room.

What To Do If Your Asthma Worsens

From "What to Do if your Asthma Worsens," reprinted with permission from the Asthma Society of Canada, © 2009. All rights reserved. For additional information about asthma, visit http://www.asthma.ca.

When you have asthma, your symptoms can vary from time to time and situation to situation. It can be difficult to know when changes in your symptoms are normal, and when they might mean trouble.

That's why it is recommended that you work with your doctor to create a written asthma action plan. Print it out and take it with you to your next doctor's appointment. Together, you can modify it as needed so that you always know when a change in your symptoms means something serious.

The Three Asthma Zones

The Green Zone—Total Asthma Control: When you're in the green zone, you have no symptoms. You're able to participate in normal activities, including strenuous physical activity. You are able to attend school or work and are sleeping through the night without asthma symptoms. You are not needing to use your reliever medication four or more times a week for asthma symptoms (except one dose prior to exercise).

Being in the green zone means your asthma is totally controlled. Continue to take your controller medications as directed by your doctor or discuss decreasing the dose if you are in the green zone more than three months. Do not stop your controller medication without first talking to your doctor.

The Yellow Zone—Warning, Loss Of Control: If you find that any of the following occur, you are in the yellow zone:

- You have asthma symptoms during regular activities or exercise.

- Your asthma symptoms begin to disturb your sleep.

- You get a cold or other chest infection.

- You need to take your reliever medication four or more times a week.

- You have missed work or school due to asthma symptoms.

If you are in the yellow zone, talk to your doctor. Your doctor will modify your medications.

The Red Zone—Emergency: Most asthma attacks are not sudden, and can be treated while in the yellow zone. However, if you are experiencing the following severe asthma symptoms, you are in the red zone and you need to get medical attention **immediately**. Make sure you recognize red zone signs:

- Excessive coughing

- Excessive wheezing

- Extreme tightness in the chest

- Extremely labored breathing

- Sweating

- Gasping voice

- Pale or blue lips or fingernails

- Anxiety or fear

- Decreased activity level

- Reliever medication does not seem to be working to relieve the symptoms

Important Phone Numbers

If any of the above symptoms are present, call 911 immediately. Have the following written down and kept close at hand in case of an emergency:

- Your doctor's name and phone number

- Local emergency service phone number

- Local ambulance service phone number

👉 **Remember!!**

Remember, it's better to be safe than sorry. To delay getting medical help when you're in the red zone can mean unnecessary suffering, even death. Always follow your action plan and your doctor's advice about how best to manage your asthma.

Source: © 2009 Asthma Society of Canada.

At The Emergency Department

If you have to go to the emergency department of a hospital, doctors and health care professionals will treat you by:

- Giving you oral or intravenous corticosteroids

- Giving you inhaled reliever medication (bronchodilator) and oxygen

- Assess your progress with spirometry, peak flow monitoring, and oximetry

Part Six

Asthma Research

Chapter 54

The National Asthma Control Program

Public Health Response To Control Asthma

As the prevalence of asthma increased during the 1980s and 1990s, federal health agencies responded. The National Asthma Education and Prevention Program (NAEPP) of the National Institutes of Health's National Heart, Lung, and Blood Institute first issued guidelines for the diagnosis and management of asthma in 1991. These guidelines translated advances in scientific and clinical research into practical advice for people with asthma, for the health care providers who look after them, and for the communities where they live.

The guidelines included the best scientific evidence about comprehensive, long-term management strategies designed to prevent and reverse airway inflammation and to manage asthma attacks. They set up standard methods for doctors to gauge the severity of a patient's asthma and monitor treatment progress. The guidelines also noted that people with asthma should use a written action plan with treatment instructions to control their illness and handle worsening asthma. They encouraged partnerships among individuals with asthma, families, and clinicians. They also laid out control measures to avoid or eliminate environmental factors that bring on asthma symptoms or attacks.

About This Chapter: Text in this chapter is excerpted from "America Breathing Easier," National Asthma Control Program, Centers for Disease Control and Prevention (CDC), 2008.

The NAEPP guidelines were updated in 1997 and 2007 to reflect new research findings, but they marked only the beginning of America's road to breathing easier. While caring for individual patients is a crucial step, the road does not end in a doctor's office or hospital. Decreasing the burden of asthma also demands a comprehensive and coordinated public health approach. That's where Centers for Disease Control and Prevention (CDC) and its partners come in.

In 1998 a group of CDC staff and federal, state, and other scientists recognized that more needed to be known about asthma if it was to be better controlled. For these professionals, the key to asthma control was surveillance—identifying and tracking asthma cases. They wanted to know:

1. How many people have asthma? How many cases occur over time?

2. What groups suffer most from asthma?

3. How severe are the cases?

4. How well are asthma cases controlled?

5. What is the cost of asthma?

CDC created the National Asthma Control Program in 1999 to launch this public health approach to asthma.

Asthma Control Program Goals And How The Program Works

Like the Healthy People 2010 goals, the asthma control program goals seek to reduce the number of deaths, hospitalizations, emergency department visits, school days or workdays missed, and limitations on activity due to asthma.

Meeting those goals means knowing the scale of the problem and having programs to help manage the problem. CDC's asthma control program has three parts: surveillance, interventions, and partnerships.

Surveillance (or tracking) lets us know how many people have asthma, where they live, and how those numbers change with the passage of time. CDC conducts surveillance activities at both the national level and, in cooperation with partners, the state level.

✎ What's It Mean?
What is surveillance?

Surveillance, also called "tracking," is the study of the distribution and occurrence of a disease in a population over time. To understand those patterns, researchers can record data such as the number of people with asthma, the number of people who go to hospitals or emergency rooms for treatment, the number of people that die from the disease, and other information.

Unlike many infectious diseases, asthma is not usually reported to the CDC, and there is no laboratory test to diagnose it. That makes it hard to know for sure how many first-time cases of asthma occur each year.

To fill in that gap, CDC uses several surveys to gather asthma information. In fact, most of what we know about how asthma affects Americans comes from surveys.

In 1999, CDC's nationwide Behavioral Risk Factor Surveillance System (BRFSS) added questions about asthma control and medication use. More detailed asthma management and control data are collected in 37 states through the National Asthma Survey, a follow-up to BRFSS.

CDC's National Health Interview Survey (NHIS) collects data on how often asthma causes days of restricted activity, days lost at work or school, physician visits, and hospitalizations.

CDC also helps states and localities collect and analyze data to better understand who gets asthma, how severe it is, and where people with asthma live, work, or go to school. This information is then used to plan and evaluate asthma interventions.

Interventions apply methods used to prevent or treat asthma. CDC conducts interventions in cooperation with state and city health officials, nongovernmental organizations, and others.

Partnerships include alliances CDC builds with states, localities, nonprofit organizations, and other federal agencies to reduce the burden of asthma.

Together, the CDC asthma control program and its many partners make up the public health response to asthma control. That response is a complex web of activities and partnerships at the national, state, and local levels. CDC provides critical support—through funding and technical guidance—to state health departments and local entities to ensure that asthma control and management are available to those in need.

State And Local Asthma Control And CDC

Partnerships between CDC and state health departments, cities, and other local entities (such as schools and nonprofit organizations) are essential for the success of asthma control in the U.S. Programs at these levels allow for more efficient use of special expertise, increased flexibility, and faster starts for programs.

♣ **It's A Fact!!**
National Healthy People 2010 Goals

• Reduce asthma deaths

• Reduce hospital emergency department visits

• Reduce number of school days or workdays missed due to asthma

• Increase the proportion of people with asthma who receive appropriate care

• Establish asthma surveillance in 15 states

Building State Capacity

CDC grants support asthma programs in 33 states, Washington, D.C., and Puerto Rico. These grants help state health departments build their asthma programs, bolster surveillance, implement interventions, and foster partnerships. In turn, this robust state capacity enhances the national public health infrastructure for addressing asthma.

Using CDC grants, 22 states have supplied training and tool kits to teach health care providers better ways to diagnose, treat, and manage asthma. Twenty three states have developed similar materials to educate school personnel so they can do more to help students control their asthma.

Building Local Programs

Cities: In 2001, CDC began to fund inner-city collaborations as part of the Controlling Asthma in American Cities Project (CAACP) with the goal of developing comprehensive and intensive community asthma control plans. Seven metropolitan areas were funded as part of CAACP: Chicago, Minneapolis/St. Paul, New York City, Oakland, Philadelphia, Richmond, and St. Louis. These projects translated existing asthma reduction strategies into services for children living in difficult social and physical environments. Based on their experience in CAACP, project staffs also created new interventions tailored to local conditions. CAACP resulted in extensive partnerships involving every level of the health care system from daycare providers to doctors.

Some programs educated daycare providers and parents about managing asthma in young children. Others integrated asthma self-management training into existing social service or faith-based organizations. One program linked high-risk children to specialty asthma services through their schools, while another worked with managed care plans to ensure reimbursement for self-management training. Some CAACP programs trained community pharmacists to educate people with asthma about using asthma medications properly, while others taught doctors the latest medical management techniques and better ways to communicate them to parents of kids with asthma.

Another successful program taught parents of children with asthma how to use diaries to make note of peak airflow, triggers, symptoms, medications, and side effects. The study coordinator then used these asthma diaries to demonstrate how long-term controller medicines worked better than rescue/quick-relief drugs in preventing asthma symptoms. The evidence in their own diaries persuaded individuals with asthma to overcome their reliance on rescue drugs.

CDC granted additional funds to CAACP cities in 2003 to implement plans like these over the next five years. The CAACP project ended in June 2008, but data collection, evaluation, and outcome studies are ongoing. In the meantime, local CAACP sites have found their own funding sources to sustain asthma control work.

Schools: As part of its Coordinated School Health Program, CDC's Division of Adolescent and School Health (DASH) implements a school-based asthma management program with the goal of increasing the number of asthma-friendly schools across the nation. Asthma-friendly schools provide a safe and supportive learning environment for students and have policies and programs in place to help students keep their asthma under good control.

DASH currently funds 10 urban school districts to implement comprehensive school asthma programs aimed at reducing student asthma episodes and absences. These school districts implement policies and programs related to improved school health services, asthma education for students and staff, and environmental management. DASH funded six national nongovernmental organizations (NGOs) from 2000–2006 to develop tools and training programs to support teachers, school nurses, school administrators, pediatricians, school board members, community members, and parents in better understanding asthma and what they can do to improve asthma management in

♣ **It's A Fact!!**
State Surveillance

State surveillance is the indispensable link between CDC's National Asthma Control Program and state health departments.

Before 1998, cities and states did not collect asthma information uniformly. Since then, CDC funding and guidance have helped state health departments standardize detailed data collection, simplifying comparison of disease rates across jurisdictions.

CDC-funded state asthma control programs now measure adult and child prevalence, indicators of asthma control, hospitalizations, and deaths. Some states also track asthma in the Medicaid population, costs attributable to asthma, or asthma management indicators—like asthma action plans, detailed medication use, school days or workdays missed due to asthma, or emergency department visits.

schools. Two of these NGOs, the American Lung Association and the American Association of School Administrators, are receiving funding to continue implementation of their asthma tools and programs from 2006–2011.

DASH also provides surveillance tools to help states and cities track progress in improved implementation of asthma management policies and practices at the state, district, and school levels, as well as self-reported asthma prevalence among middle and high school students.

Experience shows that successful school-based asthma programs share several common factors:

- They establish strong links with asthma care clinicians to ensure continued medical care.
- They focus on the greatest need, targeting for intervention students who are the most affected by asthma at school.
- They build enthusiastic administrative support within the school, including the hiring of a full-time school nurse, to coordinate a multipronged approach to controlling asthma.

Nongovernmental Organizations: CDC also works with nonprofit and health care professional organizations, including the American Lung Association; the Allergy and Asthma Foundation of America; the American Academy of Asthma, Allergy and Immunology; Allergy and Asthma Network/ Mothers of Asthmatics; and the American Thoracic Society. Safe and effective programs developed by two of these organizations are now being implemented by 12 CDC grantees—including large hospital systems, urban hospitals, city health departments, school systems, and local chapters of national asthma organizations.

The Allergy and Asthma Foundation of America's "Asthma Care Training for Kids" (ACT for Kids) teaches children how to prevent and control their symptoms. Children learn to recognize early symptoms and know what appropriate actions to take if they appear. Parents learn to encourage children to make good decisions in caring for themselves. ACT for Kids increases asthma control compliance behaviors, decreases emergency department visits, and decreases the number of days children spend in the hospital.

In the American Lung Association's "Open Airways for Schools" (OAS), children discuss basic facts about asthma and practice relaxation exercises to calm themselves during an asthma episode. They learn to identify warning signs of an asthma attack, and then develop and practice a plan for managing it. Children learn to evaluate their symptoms, use medication properly, and practice deciding when to call for medical help. They learn about environmental triggers and staying physically active. OAS boosts school performance and self-management behaviors and lowers the number of asthma attacks.

Chapter 55

Ozone, Air Quality, And Asthma

If you have asthma, you probably understand triggers—those substances or activities that bring on breathing problems. But what if your asthma trigger is in the air you breathe? Ground-level ozone and other air pollutants can trigger worsening symptoms and asthma flare-ups. But there are steps you can take to minimize your exposure.

What Is Ozone?

Ozone is a gas that's found in both the Earth's upper and lower atmospheres. The protective ozone in the upper atmosphere is very different from the harmful ozone in the lower atmosphere. Ozone that exists naturally 10 to 30 miles (16 to 48 kilometers) above the Earth protects us all from the sun's ultraviolet (UV) rays.

But ground-level ozone is different. It's found close to Earth's surface and is a serious pollutant. It's produced when sunlight combines and reacts with chemicals produced by cars, power plants, and factories. That's why

About This Chapter: This chapter begins with "Ozone, Air Quality, and Asthma," June 2007, reprinted with permission from www.kidshealth.org. Copyright © 2007 The Nemours Foundation. This information was provided by KidsHealth, one of the largest resources online for medically reviewed health information written for parents, kids, and teens. For more articles like this one, visit www.KidsHealth.org, or www.TeensHealth.org. Additional information about asthma and air quality is cited separately in the chapter.

ground-level ozone, a main component of smog, tends to be higher in sunnier climates or during hot, still weather.

Although ground ozone levels have declined somewhat since 2000, according to the American Lung Association, 47 percent of the population of the United States live in areas with unhealthy ozone levels. This includes three million children with asthma who live in towns or cities with very high levels of ozone.

♣ **It's A Fact!!**
Ozone Alert

Lots of people in the United States—an estimated 159 million—live in places that have unhealthy levels of ozone or pollution.

Source: © 2007 Nemours Foundation.

What Are Other Pollutants?

Although ozone has received a great deal of press, it's not the only pollutant that causes poor air quality. In 2004, for the first time, the American Lung Association included not only ozone but particle pollution levels in its annual "State of the Air" report for the United States.

Particle pollution refers to tiny particles of acids (such as nitrates and sulfates), dust, dirt, smoke, soot, and droplets from aerosols that are suspended in the air we breathe. The smaller the particles, the deeper they can get into the lungs, where they cause problems.

Twenty-three percent of the population of the United States, including 1,500,000 children with asthma, live in areas with levels of particle pollution that are unhealthy year-round.

In addition to ozone and particle pollution, other pollutants include gases such as carbon monoxide, sulfur dioxide, and nitrogen dioxide. High levels of these gases can also affect lung function.

How Poor Air Quality Affects People With Asthma

Air pollution is a problem for everyone—not just people with asthma. Studies have shown that high levels of air pollution can be associated with decreased lung function and more frequent reports of respiratory symptoms. This is especially true for people who spend a lot of time outdoors.

Children may be particularly affected by pollution levels because they:

- play outdoors;

- have faster breathing rates;

- have lungs that are still developing.

But although high levels of pollution affect everyone, people with asthma are more sensitive and experience the effects more quickly and severely. Additional studies have shown that ozone, particle pollution, and other forms of air pollution worsen asthma and increase hospital visits for people with asthma. And again, it's kids with asthma who are especially vulnerable to these effects.

Pollutants in the air have the same effect on people with asthma as other triggers. They reduce lung function by inflaming the lining of the lungs. Exposure to pollutants in the air can cause flare-ups and may increase the chance of upper respiratory infections, which can worsen asthma symptoms. If allergens in the air are an asthma trigger, pollutants can make the lungs even more sensitive to them.

What You Can Do

An important aspect of managing your asthma is avoiding triggers. That means you should pay attention to pollution levels and plan accordingly when they're going to be high.

The Air Quality Index (AQI) was created by the Environmental Protection Agency (EPA) to monitor outdoor air quality. In 700 counties across the United States, it measures levels of five major air pollutants regulated by the Clean Air Act:

- Ground-level ozone

- Particle pollution

- Carbon monoxide

- Sulfur dioxide

- Nitrogen dioxide

Using a color-coded system, the Air Quality Index indicates when air quality is dangerous for you. Green or yellow are acceptable colors, and orange, purple, or maroon mean you should limit your time outdoors.

The Air Quality Index varies from season to season, from day to day, and even from morning to evening. In cities larger than 350,000 people, state and local agencies are required to report the index to the public daily. But many smaller communities report the Air Quality Index as well. In many places, the next day's index is reported, so you can make plans. You can obtain Air Quality Index information:

- from weather reports;

- in the newspaper;

- at www.airnow.gov.

✔ **Quick Tip**

On days when air quality is poor, run the air conditioning and limit your time outside. Plan any outdoor activities for early in the day—when air quality tends to be better—and avoid spending time in areas where there's a lot of traffic.

If you participate in a sport that practices outside during hot weather, you should talk to the coach about alternate arrangements, such as working out in an air-conditioned gym. Also, make sure you always have your rescue medication on hand.

Improving the air quality in your home is also a good idea. You can do this by using an air cleaner, venting all gas appliances to the outside, and avoiding wood fires in your house.

You should also talk to your doctor about increasing medication during times when air pollution is high. This can be included as part of your asthma action plan.

Source: © 2007 The Nemours Foundation.

And although you can't single-handedly solve air pollution, you can take these important steps to help improve it when the air quality is poor:

- Don't drive—share a ride, take public transportation, ride a bike, or walk.

- Don't put gas in your car until after 7 p.m.

- Avoid using outboard motors, off-road vehicles, or other gasoline-powered recreational vehicles.

- Avoid mowing your lawn or using other gasoline-powered gardening equipment until the late evening or until the air quality improves.

- Don't use paints, solvents, or varnishes that produce fumes.

- If you're barbecuing, use an electric starter instead of charcoal lighter fluid.

Research Finds New Cause Of Ozone Wheezing And Potential Treatments

National Institute of Environmental Health Sciences, News Release, February 3, 2009.

Researchers at the National Institute of Environmental Health Sciences (NIEHS), part of the National Institutes of Health, and Duke University have discovered a cause of airway irritation and wheezing after exposure to ozone, a common urban air pollutant. Using an animal model, the researchers were also able to identify several ways to stop the airways from narrowing. These findings help identify potential new targets for drugs which may eventually help physicians better treat emergency room patients suffering from wheezing, coughing, and shortness of breath.

"We found that it is not the ozone itself that causes the body to wheeze, but the way the lungs respond to ozone," said Stavros Garantziotis, M.D., principal investigator in the NIEHS Laboratory of Respiratory Biology and lead author of the paper published online this week in the *Journal of Biological Chemistry*.

"Animals exposed to ozone produced and released high amounts of a sugar known as hyaluronan," said John Hollingsworth, M.D., a pulmonologist who is an assistant professor in the Department of Medicine at Duke University Medical Center and senior author of the paper. "We found hyaluronan to be directly responsible for causing the airways to narrow and become irritated. We believe this may contribute to asthma symptoms in humans as well."

The researchers found several proteins which can mediate the hyaluronan effect and can be used as treatment targets. They were also able to block the airway responsiveness by binding the native hyaluronan away, as well as by administering a slightly modified form of hyaluronan. "Although more research is needed before these findings can be translated to humans, we are optimistic these treatment options could prove beneficial to patients," said Hollingsworth.

"This finding has real-life therapeutic implications," said Garantziotis. The researchers point out there are approximately 4,500 hospital admissions and 900,000 school absences each year attributed to ozone exposure, especially on high-ozone alert days. "We identified several new approaches to the treatment of ozone-induced airway narrowing."

"This collaborative effort exemplifies the powerful advances we can continue to make to improve human health by teaming the innovativeness of our in-house researchers with our grantees," said Linda S. Birnbaum, Ph.D., NIEHS director. "This is also a good example of how NIEHS is helping to bring a pool of creative, talented young scientists to the field of environmental health sciences."

♣ It's A Fact!!

Ozone has been estimated, in an Environmental Protection Agency analysis, to cost the United States $5 billion a year as a result of premature deaths, hospitalizations, and school absences. Inhalation of ozone can lead to irritation of the airways and increased wheezing, particularly in children and adults who have asthma and chronic obstructive lung disease. Ozone is formed in the inner atmosphere in the presence of sunlight from pollutants emitted from vehicles and other sources. Exposure occurs when people inhale air containing ozone.

Source: National Institute of Environmental Health Sciences, February 3, 2009.

American Lung Association Cautions Against Wood-Burning And Urges Cleaner Alternatives For Winter Heat

"American Lung Association Cautions Against Wood-burning and Urges Cleaner Alternatives for Winter Heat," © *2009 American Lung Association. Reprinted with permission. For more information about the American Lung Association or to support the work it does, call 800-LUNG-USA (800-586-4872) or log on to www.LungUSA.org.*

As cooler temperatures begin to mark the beginning of fall, the American Lung Association warns that the comfort of a roaring fire can be harmful to your health and have a negative impact on both indoor and outdoor air quality. Burning wood emits harmful toxins and fine particles in the air that can worsen breathing problems and lead to heart and lung disease and even early death.

"With energy costs at an all time high, we are concerned about the potential impact the increased reliance on wood burning, particularly the use of wood stoves, might have on both the environment and the families who rely primarily on this method of home heating this winter," said Bernadette Toomey President and CEO of the American Lung Association.

Wood smoke poses a special threat to people with asthma and COPD and should be actively avoided by those with lung disease. When possible, the American Lung Association strongly recommends using cleaner, less toxic sources of heat. Converting a wood-burning fireplace or stove to use either natural gas or propane will eliminate exposure to the dangerous toxins wood burning generates including dioxin, arsenic and formaldehyde.

"Wood stoves manufactured before 1995 should be replaced with one that is certified by the Environmental Protection Agency and that meets the stricter standards set by the state of Washington," noted Toomey. "Vented natural gas or certified wood and pellet stoves are suitable replacements, as is installing an electric, natural gas or propane furnace."

Although both natural gas and propane stoves are much cleaner than their wood-burning alternatives, these devices must be directly vented outside the home to reduce exposure to carbon monoxide, nitrogen oxide and other emissions produced by these energy sources. Advertising claims suggest otherwise, however the American Lung Association warns that gas and propane stoves can be a threat to any family's health without proper outdoor ventilation.

When building a fire, the American Lung Association urges homeowners to take needed steps to build a cleaner fire to reduce the level of toxic emissions. Burn only 100 percent untreated wood or manufactured fireplace logs. Wood should be purchased early in the year and be stored in a covered place for at least six months before use. This will allow the wood sufficient time to dry thoroughly and ultimately will burn more efficiently and will emit less pollution.

The American Lung Association also cautions against burning other materials such as colored paper, plastics, rubber, and trash. These items generate more harmful chemicals, increased pollution and produce less heat than untreated wood or manufactured fireplace logs.

"It is also important to comply with local burn bans and to not burn wood or other materials during these times," added Toomey. "Every single chimney and wood-burning stove can have an impact on the air quality in your home and in your community."

The American Lung Association also advises home owners to be mindful of the weather. When air is cold and still, temperature inversions trap wood smoke and other pollutants close to the ground. Wood-burning should be avoided on hazy, windless days and nights.

This section of this chapter: Reprinted with permission. © 2009 American Lung Association.

Chapter 56

Hormone Fluctuations And Asthma

Editorial Note: Although the material in this chapter addresses older women, it is still helpful for teens to be aware of these issues.

Asthma, Pregnancy, And Female Hormones

Did you know that there is a strong connection between hormones and asthma? As researchers focus specifically on women and their health issues, new information has made this connection obvious. While males are more susceptible to childhood asthma, females become more susceptible to intrinsic asthma as they go through puberty and pregnancy.

In many cases menstruation can worsen the symptoms of asthma. Reproductive hormones cause smooth muscles to spasm and tissues to swell. These physiological changes can lead to symptoms of coughing, wheezing and shortness of breath.

Menopause And Asthma Decline

The fact that asthma decreases with the decline of female reproductive hormones during menopause is a strong case for the link between these

About This Chapter: Text in this chapter begins with information from "Asthma, Pregnancy and Female Hormones," reprinted with permission from www.LungDisease Focus.com. © 2009 Morefocus Media, Inc. Additional information about hormone fluctuations and asthma is cited separately in the chapter.

hormones and asthma. Women who have asthma and elect hormone replacement therapy to relieve the symptoms of menopause, find once again the strong appearance of asthma symptoms.

Pregnancy And Asthma In Women

Many asthma symptoms are known to worsen during pregnancy. The increase in the production of reproductive hormones in women may account for this. Therefore it's important to continue taking asthma medication and monitoring its effectiveness throughout pregnancy.

> **♣ It's A Fact!!**
> **Asthma And Pregnancy Stats**
>
> During pregnancy, asthma symptoms:
>
> • improve 1/3 of the time;
>
> • remain the same 1/3 of the time;
>
> • worsen 1/3 of the time.
>
> Source: © 2009 Morefocus Media, Inc.

Asthma doesn't pose a problem in the majority of pregnancies. Avoiding common triggers and making common sense decisions can help prevent the onset of asthma symptoms and attacks. Quitting smoking or avoiding situations that involve cigarette smoke is an important step in asthma maintenance for the asthmatic pregnant woman and her fetus. Research shows that cigarette smoke can harm the fetus and lead to lung impairment of the newborn.

Asthma Medication In Pregnancy

Asthmatic women are often reluctant to take the proper medication during pregnancy because of a fear of hurting the fetus. And while doctors do recommend that asthmatic women take more care with their normal asthma management routine while pregnant, most women are advised to continue taking prescribed asthma medications.

Studies suggest that most prescribed asthma medications are generally safe for the fetus. In fact, the risk of complications for a pregnant woman and her baby can be higher if asthma medication is avoided. Asthma can reduce the amount of oxygen in the mother's blood thus compromising the oxygen levels in the fetus. Premature births, low birth weight and increased maternal blood pressure are complications that can result from uncontrolled asthma. Consult your physician for specific recommendations.

While it is important for women to maintain use of their asthma medication as needed during pregnancy, it's also important to avoid unnecessary medications. A few drugs should be avoided altogether; these include adrenaline (except when prescribed by a doctor), codeine, potassium iodide, phenobarbitone and other barbiturates, tetracycline, ciprofloxacin and aminoglycoside antibiotics.

Hormone Fluctuations May Explain Higher Asthma Rates In Women

Hormone fluctuations resulting from life cycle changes are a factor in higher rates of asthma, more frequent emergency department visits, and higher hospital admission rates in women than in men according to reports at the annual meeting of the American College of Allergy, Asthma and Immunology (ACAAI) in Anaheim.

"Since we began observing a correlation between women's hormonal status and asthma symptom patterns, investigators are studying asthma incidence and mortality in relation to premenstrual and perimenstrual cycles," said Nancy K. Ostrom, M.D., at the University of California and the Allergy & Asthma Medical Group and Research Center in San Diego.

"Women between the ages of 20–50 years are more than three times as likely as men to be hospitalized with asthma despite comparable spirometry. Studies have demonstrated a relationship between asthma and the menstrual cycle, with 46 percent of women's hospital admissions perimenstrual, and up to 40 percent of women having premenstrual asthma symptoms," Dr. Ostrom said.

"As many as 8 percent of pregnant women have asthma. Women with asthma who are pregnant or are planning a pregnancy face unique concerns about controlling their asthma symptoms and regarding the safety of medications," she said.

Obesity, sedentary lifestyle, and smoking are other factors potentially contributing to the gender difference in asthma morbidity and mortality according to Dr. Ostrom.

"When we look at the reproductive phases of a woman's life cycle, we find in children under age 12, asthma is more common in boys than in girls. Around puberty the ratio changes, with asthma becoming more common in girls than in boys. Asthma is three times more common in women than in men," said Joan Gluck, M.D., at the Florida Center for Allergy and Asthma Care in Miami.

"Women with asthma experience more symptoms during their premenstrual and menstrual weeks with peak symptoms two to three days before menses. Many are not aware of this pattern, and keeping a diary of their symptoms is very helpful," she said.

Most premenstrual asthma patients respond to standard therapy. Some need increased inhaled corticosteroids or long-acting beta-agonist (LABA) on days 19–4 of their cycle [that is, the 19th day of one cycle through the 4th day of the next cycle]. A small subset of women are unresponsive to the usual therapy. Oral contraceptives have been shown to have an impact on asthma.

"Nonasthmatic women on oral contraceptives have a higher total lung capacity. Airways are more stable in women with asthma who take oral contraceptives, and several small studies have shown their asthma does improve," Dr. Gluck said.

A correlation with higher asthma rates has also been noted in menopause and perimenopause, occurring prior to final menstrual cycle.

"Hormone replacement therapy (HRT) has different effects on asthma for different groups. Nonasthmatic women taking HRT have a higher risk of developing asthma. However, asthmatic women significantly improve on HRT, with studies showing as much as a 35 percent reduction in the use of inhaled steroids," Dr. Gluck said.

Asthma complicates up to 8 percent of pregnancies and may increase the risk of perinatal complications according to Michael Schatz, M.D., M.S., at Kaiser-Permanente Medical Center in San Diego, California.

When women with asthma become pregnant, a third of the patients improve, one third worsen, and the last third remain unchanged. Asthma exacerbations are most likely to appear during the weeks 24 to 36 of gestation, with only a small minority of patients (20 percent or fewer) becoming symptomatic during labor and delivery.

"Patients with more severe asthma prior to pregnancy may be more likely to worsen during pregnancy. Uncontrolled asthma may increase the risk of perinatal mortality, low birth weight infants, preterm births and preeclampsia," Dr. Schatz said.

Management of asthma during pregnancy includes assessment and monitoring; reduction of triggers, patient education, and pharmacologic therapy. Optimal management of asthma during pregnancy minimizes the risks, and improves maternal and fetal outcomes. Poor asthma control is the major risk to the health of the mother and fetus.

"A recent study demonstrated that asthma may be under-treated in women who are pregnant and who are contemplating pregnancy. For patients using inhaled corticosteroids (ICS) before pregnancy, the rate of asthma-related physician visits decreased and the number of emergency department (ED) visits was unchanged after pregnancy. Physician and ED visits increased after pregnancy for patients not using an ICS before pregnancy," Dr. Schatz said.

According to recent National Asthma Education and Prevention Program guidelines, ICS are recommended as the controller therapy of choice for all levels of persistent asthma during pregnancy. Because of more reassuring data, inhaled budesonide is the preferred ICS for use during pregnancy, although other ICS may be continued in patients well-controlled on them prior to pregnancy.

Medications to be avoided during pregnancy include epinephrine (except for anaphylaxis), iodides, certain antibiotics, prostaglandin F2 analogues, ergonovine, and methylergonovine.

"Although the outcome of any pregnancy can never be guaranteed, most women with asthma and allergies do well with proper medical management by physicians familiar with these disorders and the changes that occur during pregnancy," Dr. Schatz said.

Chapter 57

New Treatments For Asthma

New Treatments Improve Control For Severe Asthma

Over just one decade, new asthma medications and tools have significantly improved the management of this serious airway disease.

When compared to children treated in the mid-90s, children with severe asthma during 2004 to 2007 were less likely to need oral steroids and rescue inhalers, and their lung function scores were improved, according to a study from National Jewish Health in Denver.

"The current cohort was less likely to require chronic oral glucocorticoids, have better asthma control, and have fewer glucocorticoid-induced adverse effects compared to a cohort of severe asthmatic children studied a decade ago," wrote the authors.

Results of the study were presented at the American Academy of Allergy, Asthma & Immunology (AAAAI) annual meeting, in Washington, D.C.

To assess whether or not newer medications such as newer inhaled steroids, combinations of inhaled steroids and long-acting bronchodilators

(Advair), and leukotriene receptor antagonists (Singulair) had made a positive impact on asthma treatment, the researchers compared a group of 65 children referred to the hospital between 2004 and 2007 to 164 children who were referred to National Jewish between 1993 and 1997. All of the children had severe asthma.

Just over three quarters of the present-day group were on a leukotriene receptor antagonist, and two-thirds were on combination medication. None of the group from the 90s took any of these medications.

Compared to the historic group, the present-day children were less likely to need oral steroids—28 percent of the current group versus 51 percent of the historic group. When oral steroids were needed, the present-day group required only about one-quarter of the dose that was required 10 years earlier.

Today's group turned to their rescue (albuterol) inhaler about half as often as the group from the 90s did, and their lung function scores were higher. They also required less intubations than did children in the past—13 percent versus 21 percent.

"The medication playing the greatest role in this improvement to date is inhaled corticosteroids," said Dr. Alissa Hersh, an assistant clinical professor in the division of allergy and immunology at Morgan Stanley Children's Hospital of New York-Presbyterian in New York City. "If we can keep them on preventive medications, we can keep them from having acute exacerbations."

Dr. Jennifer Appleyard, chief of allergy and immunology at St. John Hospital in Detroit, agreed that inhaled steroids are the most effective first-line treatment. However, she also pointed out that the U.S. National Institutes of Health first issued their asthma management guidelines in the mid-90s, and she said that guidance has likely played a role in improved asthma management as well.

Appleyard said she wished the authors had also looked at hospitalization and death rates to see if there were any differences.

"Newer medications are much more effective in treating people with severe asthma, but this doesn't mean the battle is over. People are still dying from asthma," she said.

One problem may be compliance with the doctor's orders when it comes to taking medications. A second study that was expected to be presented at the same meeting found that even when people have insurance, and they have a regular doctor, they may not always follow their asthma management plans. The study found that about one in four children with insurance were using inhaled corticosteroids while just one in five uninsured children were. The published study information did not identify the severity of the asthma.

Another study, this one from the Agency for HealthCare Research and Quality, suggests that insurance status does affect compliance. This study found that 30 percent of those with insurance were taking preventive asthma medications, while only 18 percent without insurance were on the drugs.

"We've made a significant impact on asthma management, and we're definitely moving in the right direction," said Hersh, who added, "The ultimate goal is not just to prevent asthma, but ultimately to find a cure."

New Approach To Treating Asthma Suggested

From "New Approach to Treating Asthma Suggested," February 15, 2009. © 2009 Texas Medical Center. Reprinted with permission.

Stimulants have long been used to treat asthma, but a new research study has motivated a University of Houston (UH) professor to suggest that an opposite approach to asthma treatment may be in order.

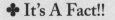

♣ It's A Fact!!

Beta blockers work to block the actions of receptors that receive and respond to stimuli in the smooth muscle that lines the airways. Stimulants, on the other hand, stimulate the receptors in hope of reducing asthma symptoms.

Source: © 2009 Texas Medical Center.

Richard Bond, Ph.D., professor of pharmacology at UH's College of Pharmacy, has been investigating whether beta blockers could be safer and more effective for treating long-term asthma than stimulants—the current method of treatment.

A recent study published in the online journal *Proceedings of the*

National Academy of Sciences showed that mice without the gene that produces the receptors have no asthma-like symptoms. In other words, mice without the receptors have no asthma-like symptoms. This led Bond to question whether the pharmaceutical industry should be working to block or inhibit the receptor, instead of stimulating it to reduce asthma symptoms.

The timely release of this study comes on the heels of the U.S. Food and Drug Administration (FDA) considering a renewed look at the use of stimulants, some of which have been associated with increased risk of hospitalization and asthma-related deaths.

Bond's proposal to use beta blockers instead of stimulants is an approach termed "paradoxical pharmacology," meaning that the beta blockers may initially worsens patients' symptoms before eventually improving their overall health.

Beta blockers currently are contraindicated for asthma because they typically trigger bronchoconstriction, decreasing the flow of air to the lungs. Bond has suggested, however, that although beta blockers would not replace the need for emergency inhalers for acute episodes, the negative effects associated with beta blockers eventually taper off to provide long-term relief from asthma symptoms. In addition, several studies have shown chronic use of stimulants cause the body to become desensitized to the stimulants, thereby rendering them ineffective against asthma.

With support from the Strategic Program for Asthma Research of the American Asthma Foundation, a second human clinical trial based on Bond's research is under way using the beta-blocker drug nadolol in patients with mild asthma.

A first human trial gained support for beta blockers. In commenting on the trial, two British researchers wrote in the January 10 [2009] issue of the British medical journal *The Lancet* that "the use of beta-blocker therapy for asthma warrants . . . consideration and further investigation . . ."

To those ends, a company called Inverseon, of which Bond is scientific founder, has filed U.S. patent applications for using beta blockers to treat airway disease. William Garner, chairman of Inverseon, said the company recently received a notice of allowance—one of several procedural steps on the path to patent approval—from the U.S. Patent Office.

Bronchial Thermoplasty And Asthma Treatment

"Bronchial Thermoplasty and Asthma Treatment," reprinted with permission from www.LungDiseaseFocus.com. © 2009 Morefocus Media, Inc.

Bronchial thermoplasty is a potential new asthma treatment currently undergoing clinical testing. Developed by Asthmatx, Inc. (a medical device company), bronchial thermoplasty has the potential to provide asthma relief to people who do not respond to conventional asthma treatment.

The *American Journal of Respiratory and Critical Care Medicine* reported results of a small bronchial thermoplasty clinical trial in it's May 2006 edition. The study monitored sixteen adults with mild to moderate asthma that did not respond to current asthma treatments for two years after receiving bronchial thermoplasty treatment.

Bronchial Thermoplasty Treatment

Bronchial thermoplasty uses radio frequency energy to relieve asthma symptoms. Because the procedure requires only light anesthesia, it can be performed on an outpatient basis. A small, flexible tube called a bronchoscope is inserted through the nose or mouth and guided into the lungs.

♣ It's A Fact!!
Clinical Trial Results

The results of the small bronchial thermoplasty study are encouraging. Two years after bronchial thermoplasty treatment, 75 percent of the participants reported that the asthma treatment allowed them to function better in daily activities.

Participants also reported:

- an increase in symptom-free days;

- less difficulty with asthma triggers;

- reduced peak expiratory flow readings.

Bronchial thermoplasty appears to be a well-tolerated asthma treatment, with minimal side effects. Almost all participants said they would be willing to undergo the asthma treatment a second time.

Source: © 2009 Morefocus Media, Inc.

Once the bronchoscope is situated in the desired airway, a catheter is inserted through the bronchoscope. The tip of the catheter is inflated until it touches the sides of the airway wall. Radio frequency energy is then sent through the catheter, heating the smooth muscle walls of the airway to approximately 149 degrees F. This temperature is sufficient to thin the smooth airway wall muscles without scarring or damaging them.

During an asthma attack, the smooth muscles of the airways contract. Because bronchial thermoplasty thins the muscle walls, they cannot narrow as much when irritants trigger asthma attacks, resulting in less symptoms and asthma relief. Participants in the bronchial thermoplasty study received three thirty-minute thermoplasty treatments that treated all accessible airways.

What's Next For Bronchial Thermoplasty?

With such promising initial results, bronchial thermoplasty is receiving some attention as a possible new asthma treatment. The sixteen volunteers from the small clinical study will be monitored for an additional five years. Studies on the effectiveness of bronchial thermoplasty are ongoing: two larger bronchial thermoplasty studies ended in 2006. Similarly, a fourth study has begun that will monitor 300 participants at over 30 international medical centers.

Asthmatx Inc. points out that bronchial thermoplasty is an alternative to conventional asthma treatment. While the procedure is designed to reduce asthma symptoms, it is not intended to serve as a cure for the disease.

Simpler Asthma Treatment Options Found Effective

Excerpted from "Simpler Asthma Treatment Options Found Effective," © 2009 American Lung Association. Reprinted with permission. For more information about the American Lung Association or to support the work it does, call 800-LUNG-USA (800-586-4872) or log on to www.LungUSA.org.

American Lung Association Clinical Trial Tested Specific Drugs Head-To-Head With Gold Standard Of Asthma Treatment

Results of American Lung Association clinical research published today in the *New England Journal of Medicine* found that a simpler, once-a-day regimen of a combination inhaler containing an inhaled corticosteroid and a long-acting beta-agonist is just as effective as twice-daily inhaled cortico-steroid treatment in patients with mild persistent asthma, which may open the doors to more convenient treatment plans for millions of Americans.

"For patients, a simpler treatment plan means less drugs to take—and to remember to take—every day, fewer prescription refills and perhaps less money spent on medications, and fewer side effects. This is the kind of practical research that is helpful immediately for both physicians and patients alike."

"It's certainly easier to do something once a day rather than twice a day," said Stephen P. Peters, MD, PhD, lead author of the study and Professor of Medicine and Pediatrics, Wake Forest University School of Medicine. "Now physicians can discuss reasonable alternatives for step-down treatment for patients who gain asthma control with standard therapy based on solid evidence from a randomized controlled clinical trial, which is the best way to evaluate and compare treatment alternatives."

Reprinted with permission. © 2009 American Lung Association.

Chapter 58

Medicines That Can Make Asthma Worse

Why should I be careful about taking medicine if I have asthma?

Certain medicines might aggravate your asthma and make it worse. Not all people who have asthma experience problems when taking these medicines. However, if you have asthma, it's important to know about medicines that might cause problems before you take them.

Will aspirin and other pain relievers make my asthma worse?

Aspirin and other drugs called non-steroidal anti-inflammatory drugs (NSAIDs) may be harmful in people who have asthma. Ibuprofen (one brand name: Motrin), naproxen (one brand name: Aleve) and ketoprofen (one brand name: Orudis) are a few examples of non-steroidal anti-inflammatory drugs. If you are allergic to aspirin, ask your doctor or pharmacist to make sure any new medicine you might take is not related to aspirin.

Acetaminophen (one brand name: Tylenol) can usually be taken safely by people who have asthma. This medicine is typically used to relieve fever and pain. Very rarely, even acetaminophen may make asthma worse. If this happens to you, tell your doctor. He or she can help you find another type of reliever.

About This Chapter: Reprinted with permission from "Asthma: Medicines That Can Make It Worse," September 2003. Updated September 2008, http://familydoctor.org/online/famdocen/home/common/asthma/medications/171.html. Copyright © 2008 American Academy of Family Physicians. All Rights Reserved.

♣ It's A Fact!!
Acetaminophen May Increase The Risk Of Developing Asthma

There is a growing body of scientific literature suggesting a causal link between the use of the non-steroidal anti-inflammatory drug acetaminophen and the rise in the incidence of asthma in children. A new epidemiologic study, supported by the National Institute of Environmental Health Sciences (NIEHS), conducted with 345 pregnant women adds to the growing evidence.

There are plausible biological and associative links between acetaminophen and asthma. Acetaminophen became the drug of choice for pain and fever relief in the 1980s after several studies reported a link between Reye syndrome and aspirin use. In 1986, the FDA placed warning labels regarding the Reye syndrome link on acetaminophen bottles. Shortly afterwards, pediatricians nationwide started noticing a rise in asthma incidence. Acetaminophen, unlike aspirin and ibuprofen, decreases the level of the antioxidant glutathione in the lungs and other tissues.

In the NIEHS-funded work, women were recruited during their first trimester of pregnancy. Use of acetaminophen during pregnancy was determined by a questionnaire and related to respiratory outcomes in their newborns during their first year of life. Use of acetaminophen in the second and third trimesters was significantly related to wheezing in the first year. While wheezing is a known symptom of asthma in young children, it alone does not constitute a diagnosis of asthma.

The findings in this report are consistent with previous literature showing increases in asthma symptoms after exposure to acetaminophen. The researchers will continue to follow these children until they reach five years of age, enabling them to provide more precise estimates of asthma incidence. The researchers point out that this is only the second study suggesting that exposure to acetaminophen late in pregnancy may affect the subsequent development of allergic symptoms in the child. Confirmation of these finding in larger cohorts could have substantial public health implications in defining factors attributable to the development of asthma.

Source: National Institute of Environmental Health Sciences, November 2008.

Can I take antihistamines for my allergies?

Antihistamines are usually safe for people who have asthma to use, but they can cause side effects. Some antihistamines can't be taken with certain other medicines. Like any other medicine, read the warnings and instructions on the label and check with your doctor before you start taking an antihistamine.

What about medicines for blood pressure?

Beta-blockers, used to control blood pressure and heart disease, can make asthma worse. This group of drugs includes propranolol (brand name: Inderal), atenolol (brand name: Tenormin) and metoprolol (brand names: Lopressor, Toprol). If you have started taking a beta-blocker and your asthma gets worse, tell your doctor.

Angiotensin-converting enzyme (ACE) inhibitors are another type of medicine given to treat blood pressure, heart disease and, sometimes, diabetes. Drugs such as captopril (brand name: Capoten), enalapril (brand name: Vasotec) and lisinopril (brand names: Prinivil, Zestril) are included in this group. These medicines appear to be safe for people who have asthma. However, some people develop a cough when taking ACE inhibitors.

If you start coughing while you're taking an ACE inhibitor, remember that the cough might not be caused by your asthma. If the cough is caused by the ACE inhibitor, it will usually go away a week or so after you stop taking it. If you develop other problems that make your asthma worse, call your doctor to see if you should stop taking your ACE inhibitor.

What about contrast dye for x-rays?

Sometimes when you have an x-ray, you have to drink or get an injection of contrast dye to make the x-ray picture show up. Some contrast dyes may trigger an asthma attack. It's very important that you tell your doctor or the x-ray technician that you have asthma. Sometimes they can give you another medicine before you get the contrast dye, so the dye won't cause problems.

How do I know if other medicines I'm taking are making my asthma worse?

Any medicine can cause wheezing or shortness of breath if you're allergic to it. If you notice that your asthma gets worse every time you take a certain medicine, tell your doctor as soon as possible. If you use a peak flow meter to check your asthma, tell your doctor if you see changes in your peak flow readings after you take a certain medicine. Your doctor can decide if your medicine should be changed.

♣ It's A Fact!!
Asthma And Wheeze In Young Women Taking Oral Contraceptives

Oral contraceptive use by young women may influence the occurrence of asthma and wheezing according to research performed at the University of Southern California Keck School of Medicine. Oral contraceptive use was associated with about an 80 percent reduction in wheezing, a sign of a flare up of the disease, in women with a history of asthma.

Previous research by this group and others has shown that sex steroid hormones may play a role in asthma. To expand on this body of research, this NIEHS-supported team conducted an epidemiologic study in a population of 905 women aged 13–28. The results were somewhat variable depending on the whether women had a history of asthma. In women without asthma, oral contraceptive use was associated with a 75 percent increase in the prevalence of wheeze. And women who reached puberty before age twelve were twice as likely to develop asthma after puberty.

The age at which girls reach puberty has been declining in the same time period that asthma prevalence has been increasing. The authors conclude that sex hormones may play an important role in asthma occurrence. Oral contraceptive use and asthma are common among young women; therefore, these findings are likely to have public health implications. The authors also suggest that clinicians may want to inform young women about the potential effects of oral contraceptive use on asthma-related respiratory symptoms.

Source: National Institute of Environmental Health Sciences, May 2006.

Part Seven

If You Need Additional Help And Information

Chapter 59

Asthma Organizations

Allergy and Asthma Network Mothers of Asthmatics
2751 Prosperity Avenue, Suite 150
Fairfax, VA 22031
Toll Free: (800) 878-4403
Fax: (703) 573-7794
Website: http://www.aanma.org

Allies Against Asthma
Center for Managing Chronic Disease
University of Michigan
School of Public Health
109 Observatory Street
Ann Arbor, MI 48109-2029
Phone: (734) 615-3312
Fax: (734) 763-9115
Website: http://
www.asthma.umich.edu
E-mail: asthma@umich.edu

American Academy of Allergy, Asthma, and Immunology
555 East Wells Street, Suite 1100
Milwaukee, WI 53202-3823
Phone: (414) 272-6071
Website: http://www.aaaai.org
E-mail: info@aaaai.org

American Academy of Family Physicians
11400 Tomahawk Creek Parkway
Leawood, KS 66211-2680
Phone: (913) 906-6000
Toll Free: (800) 274-2237
Fax: (913) 906-6075
Website: http://www.aafp.org

About This Chapter: Information in this chapter was compiled from many sources deemed accurate; inclusion does not constitute endorsement. All contact information verified in August 2009.

American Academy of Pediatrics

141 Northwest Point Boulevard
Elk Grove Village, IL 60007-1098
Phone: (847) 434-4000
Fax: (847) 434-8000
Website: http://www.aap.org
E-mail: kidsdocs@aap.org

American Association for Respiratory Care

9425 North MacArthur Boulevard
Suite 100
Irving, TX 75063-4706
Phone: (972) 243-2272
Website: http://www.aarc.org
E-mail: info@aarc.org

American College of Allergy, Asthma, and Immunology

85 West Algonquin Road
Suite 550
Arlington Heights, IL 60005
Phone: (847) 427-1200
Fax: (847) 427-1294
Website: http://www.acaai.org
E-mail: mail@acaai.org

American College of Chest Physicians

3300 Dundee Road
Northbrook, IL 60062-2348
Phone: (847) 498-1400
Toll Free: (800) 343-2227
Website: http://www.chestnet.org

American Lung Association

1301 Pennsylvania Avenue, NW
Suite 800
Washington, DC 20004
Referral to the ALA closest to you:
(800) 586-4872
To speak with a lung health
professional: (800) 548-8252
National headquarters:
(212) 315-8700
Website: http://www.lungusa.org

American Rhinologic Society

P.O. Box 495
Warwick, NY 10990-0495
Phone: (845) 988-1631
Fax: (845) 986-1527
Website: http://
www.american-rhinologic.org
E-mail: arsinfo
@american-rhinologic.org

Association of Occupational and Environmental Clinics

1010 Vermont Avenue, NW #513
Washington, DC 20005
Phone: (202) 347-4976
Toll Free: (888) 347-2632
Fax: (202) 347-4950
Website: http://www.aoec.org
E-mail: aoec@aoec.org

Asthma and Allergy Foundation of America

8201 Corporate Drive, Suite 1000
Landover, MD 20785
Phone: (800) 727-8462
Website: http://www.aafa.org
E-mail: Info@aafa.org

The Asthma Center Education and Research Fund

205 North Broad Street, Suite 300
Philadelphia, PA 19107
Phone: (215) 569-1111
Website: http://
www.theasthmacenter.org

Asthma Initiative of Michigan

403 Seymour
Lansing, MI 48933
Phone: (866) 395-8647 (MI only)
Phone: (517) 484-7206
Website: http://
www.getasthmahelp.org
E-mail: info@GetAsthmaHelp.org

Asthma Society of Canada

4950 Yonge Street, Suite 2306
Toronto, Ontario M2N 6K1
Canada
Phone: (416) 787-4050
(for Toronto residents)
Toll Free: (866) 787-4050
(for Canadian residents)
Fax: (416) 787-5807
Website: http://www.asthma.ca
E-mail: info@asthma.ca

Canadian Centre for Occupational Health and Safety

135 Hunter Street East
Hamilton, Ontario L8N 1M5
Canada
Phone: (905) 572-2981
Fax: (905) 572-2206
Website: http://www.ccohs.ca

Canadian Lung Association

1750 Courtwood Crescent
Suite 300
Ottawa, Ontario K2C 2B5
Canada
Phone: (613) 569-6411
Toll Free: (888) 566-5864
Fax: (613) 569-8860
Website: http://www.lung.ca
E-mail: info@lung.ca

Canadian Network for Asthma Care

16851 Mount Wolfe Road
Caledon, Ontario L7E 3P6
Canada
Phone: (905) 880-1092
Fax: (905) 880-9733
Website: http://www.cnac.net

Centers for Disease Control and Prevention

1600 Clifton Road
Atlanta, GA 30333
Toll Free: (800) 232-4636
Website: http://www.cdc.gov
E-mail: cdcinfo@cdc.gov

Children's Environmental Health Center
Mount Sinai School of Medicine
One Gustave L. Levy Place
New York, NY 10029
Phone: (212) 241-6500
Website: http://
www.childenvironment.org

Cleveland Clinic Foundation
9500 Euclid Avenue
Cleveland, OH 44195
Phone: (216) 444-2200
Toll Free: (800) 223-2273
Website: http://
my.clevelandclinic.org

Consortium on Children's Asthma Camps
490 Concordia Avenue
St. Paul, MN 55103
Phone: (651) 227-8014
Website: http://
www.asthmacamps.org

Family Allergy and Asthma
Website: http://
www.familyallergy.com

Food Allergy and Anaphylaxis Network
11781 Lee Jackson Hwy., Suite 160
Fairfax, VA 22033-3309
Toll Free: (800) 929-4040
Fax: (703) 691-2713
Website: http://
www.foodallergy.org
E-mail: faan@foodallergy.org

Food and Drug Administration
10903 New Hampshire Ave.
Silver Spring, MD 20903
Toll Free: (888) 463-6332
Website: http://www.fda.gov

Global Initiative for Asthma
Website: http://www.ginasthma.com

Healthy Kids
Phone: (617) 965-9637
Website: http://www.healthy-kids
.info
E-mail: healthykids@rcn.com

Indoor Air Quality
U.S. Environmental Protection
Agency
Office of Radiation
Indoor Environments Division
Phone: (202) 343-9370
1200 Pennsylvania Avenue, NW
Mail Code 6609J
Washington, DC 20460
Website: http://www.epa.gov/iaq

MyDr.com.au

2nd Floor, 1 Chandros Street
St. Leonards NSW 2065
Australia
Website: http://www.mydr.com.au

National Allergy Bureau

American Academy of Allergy,
Asthma, and Immunology
Executive Office
555 East Wells Street, 11th Floor
Milwaukee, WI 53202-3823
Phone: (414) 272-6071
Fax: (414) 272-6070
Website: http://www.aaaai.org/nab
E-mail: nab@aaaai.org

National Association of School Nurses

8484 Georgia Avenue, Suite 420
Silver Spring, MD 20910
Phone: (240) 821-1130
Toll Free: (866) 627-6767
Fax: (301) 585-1791
Website: http://www.nasn.org
E-mail: nasn@nasn.org

National Education Association

Health Information Network
1201 16th Street NW, Suite 216
Washington, DC 20036
Phone: (202) 822-7570
Website: http://www.neahin.org
E-mail: info@neahin.org

National Heart, Lung, and Blood Institute

Health Information Center
P.O. Box 30105
Bethesda, MD 20824-0105
Phone: (301) 592-8573
Fax: (301) 592-8563
Website: http://www.nhlbi.nih.gov/
E-mail: nhlbiinfo@nhlbi.nih.gov

National Institute of Allergy and Infectious Diseases

6610 Rockledge Drive MSC 6612
Bethesda, MD 20892-6612
Phone: (301) 496-5717
Toll Free: (866) 284-4107
Fax: (301) 402-3573
Website: http://www3.niaid.nih.gov

National Institute of Environmental Health Sciences

P.O. Box 12233, MD K3-16
Research Triangle Park,
NC 27709-2233
Phone: (919) 541-3345
Fax: (919) 541-4395
Website: http://www.niehs.nih.gov

National Jewish Health

1400 Jackson Street
Denver, CO 80206
Phone: (303) 398-1355
Toll Free: (800) 222-5864 (lung line)
Toll Free: (800) 423-8891 (hospital)
Website: http://www.nationaljewish.org

National Library of Medicine
8600 Rockville Pike
Bethesda, MD 20894
Phone: (301) 594-5983
Toll Free: (888) 346-3656
Fax: (301) 402-1384
Website: http://www.nlm.nih.gov
E-mail: custserv@nlm.nih.gov

National Lung Health Education Program
American Association for Respiratory Care
9425 MacArthur Boulevard
Irving, TX 75063
Phone: (972) 910-8555
Fax: (972) 484-2720
Website: http://www.nlhep.org
E-mail: nelson@nlhep.org

Nemours Foundation
10140 Centurion Parkway North
Jacksonville, FL 32256
Phone: (904) 697-4100
Fax: (904) 697-4125
Website: http://www.nemours.org

Pediatric/Adolescent Gastroesophageal Reflux Association (PAGER)
P.O. Box 486
Buckeystown, MD 21717-0486
Phone: (310) 601-9541
Website: http://www.reflux.org
E-mail: gergroup@aol.com

Chapter 60

If You Would Like To Read More About Asthma

Books

100 Questions and Answers About Asthma. Plotte, Claudia S. Sudbury, MA: Jones and Bartlett Publishers, Inc., 2005.

American Academy of Pediatrics Guide to Your Child's Allergies and Asthma: Breathing Easy and Bringing Up Healthy, Active Children. Welch, Michael J. and American Academy of Pediatrics. New York: Random House, 2000.

The American Lung Association Family Guide to Asthma and Allergies. The American Lung Association Asthma Advisory Group with Norman H. Edelman, M.D., New York: Little Brown and Company, 1998.

The Asthma and Allergy Action Plan for Kids: A Complete Program to Help Your Child Life a Full and Active Life. Dozor, Allen and Kate Kelly. New York: Fireside, 2004.

Asthma: The Complete Guide to Self-Management of Asthma and Allergies for Patients and Their Families. Weinstein, Allan M. Fawcett Books, 1992.

Asthma for Dummies. Berger, William E., and Jackie Joyner-Kersee. Indianapolis, IN: Wiley Publishing, Inc., 2004.

Asthma & Exercise. Hogshead, Nancy and Gerald Secor Couzens. New York: Henry Holt and Company, 1991.

Asthma: Questions You Have...Answers You Need. Casler, Kristin. New York: HarperTorch, 2000.

Asthma: Stop Suffering, Start Living, 3rd Edition. Gershwin, Eric, E. I. Klingelhofer and M. Eric Gershwin. Cambridge, MA: Da Capo Press, 2001.

Asthma: The Ultimate Teen Guide, 2nd Edition. Hutchins Paquette, Penny. Lanham, MD: The Scarecrow Press, 2006.

Breathe Easy: Young People's Guide to Asthma. Weiss, Jonathan H. and Michael Chesworth (illustrator). Washington, DC: Magination Press, 2003.

Bronchial Asthma: A Guide for Practical Understanding and Treatment. Gershwin, M. Eric and Timothy E. Albertson. Totowa, New Jersey: Humana Press, 2006.

The Complete Allergy Book: Learn to Become Actively Involved in Your Own Care. Kwong, Frank. Naperville, IL: Sourcebooks, Inc., 2002.

The Complete Kid's Allergy and Asthma Guide: Allergy and Asthma Information for Children of All Ages. Gold, Milton. Toronto, Canada: Robert Rose, Inc., 2003.

Conquering Asthma—An Illustrated Guide to Understanding and Self Care. Barnes, Peter J. and Michael T. Newhouse. Manson Publishing Ltd., 1994.

The Harvard Medical School Guide To Taking Control Of Asthma. Fanta, Christopher H., Lynda M. Cristiano and Kenan Haver. New York: Free Press, 2003.

Living Well with Asthma. Freedman, Michael R., Samuel J. Rosenberg and Cynthia L. Divino. New York: The Guilford Press, 1998.

Shortness of Breath: A Guide to Better Living and Breathing. Ries, Andrew L., et al. Mosby, 2000.

Taming Asthma and Allergy by Controlling Your Environment: A Guide for Patients. Wood, Robert A. Asthma and Allergy Foundation of America, 1995.

What To Do When The Doctor Says It's Asthma: Everything You Need to Know About Medicines, Allergies, Food and Exercise to Breath more Easily Every Day. Hannaway, Paul. Beverly, MA: Fair Winds Press, 2004.

Websites

Allergy and Asthma Network, Mothers of Asthmatics
http://www.aanma.org

American Academy of Allergy Asthma and Immunology
http://www.aaaai.org

American College of Allergy, Asthma and Immunology
http://www.acaai.org

American College of Chest Physicians
http://chestnet.org

American Lung Association
http://www.lungusa.org

Asthma and Allergy Foundation of America
http://www.aafa.org

Asthma Initiative of Michigan
http://www.getasthmahelp.org

Asthma Society of Canada
http://www.asthmakids.ca

Canadian Centre for Occupational Health and Safety

http://www.ccohs.ca

Centers for Disease Control and Prevention

http://www.cdc.gov/asthma

Cleveland Clinic

http://my.clevelandclinic.org

Family Allergy & Asthma

http://www.familyallergy.com

Global Initiative for Asthma

http://www.ginasthma.org

MyDr.com.au

http://mydr.com.au

National Institute of Allergy and Infectious Diseases

http://www3.niaid.nih.gov

National Institute of Environmental Health Sciences, National Institutes of Health

http://www.niehs.nih.gov/health/topics/conditions/asthma/index.cfm

The Nemours Foundation

http://www.kidshealth.org/teen/diseases_conditions/allergies_immune/asthma_center.html

United States Environmental Protection Agency

http://www.epa.gov

World Health Organization

http://www.who.int/en

Web-Based Documents And Resources

4 Seasons of Asthma
Asthma Society of Canada
http://www.4seasonsofasthma.ca

AIRNow
A cross-agency U.S. Government Web site
Web page for this resource: http://www.airnow.gov/

Asthma Action Plan
National Heart Lung and Blood Institute
Web page for this resource: http://www.nhlbi.nih.gov/health/public/lung/
asthma/asthma_actplan.h

Asthma Financial Assistance Program
Patient Services Incorporated
http://www.uneedpsi.org

Asthma Kids
Asthma Society of Canada
http://www.asthmakids.ca

Asthma Management and Education Online
Asthma and Allergy Foundation of America
Web page for resource: http://aafa.org/display.cfm?id=4&sub=82&cont=395

Asthma and Physical Activity in the School
National Heart Lung and Blood Institute
Web page for this resource: http://www.nhlbi.nih.gov/health/public/lung/
asthma/phy_asth.htm

Attack Asthma. Learn More.
U.S. Environmental Protection Agency
Web page for this resource: http://www.noattacks.org

Profiler Treatment Option Tool for Asthma
American Lung Association
https://www.lungprofiler.nexcura.com/Secure/
InterfaceSecure.asp?CB=26270

So You Have Asthma
National Heart Lung and Blood Institute
Web page for this resource: http://www.nhlbi.nih.gov/health/public/lung/
asthma/have_asthma.htm

Index

Index

Page numbers that appear in *Italics* refer to illustrations. Page numbers that have a small 'n' after the page number refer to information shown as Notes at the beginning of each chapter. Page numbers that appear in **Bold** refer to information contained in boxes on that page (except Notes information at the beginning of each chapter).